WHAT A *Doctor* LOOKS LIKE

Society's unrealistic dreams are your attainable goals

TAMIKA K. CROSS, MD

Published by University of Moguls Publishing and Design

Cover design by University of Moguls Publishing and Design
www.universityofmoguls.com

ISBN-13: 978-1-7366581-6-1

This book is dedicated to my late grandmother,
Jeanne Legge-Taylor.
You are my inspiration to write and my inspiration
in becoming a physician. I love and miss you.

Table of Contents

Foreword

It was summer 1987, and our family was on the road heading back from Boblo Island. Trips to Boblo were always a favorite pastime of many people in Detroit. We would board the boat and head over to the Canadian side of the Detroit river, enjoy the amusement park, and take the boat back at the end of the day. I was riding in the backseat with my baby boy, Melvin Jr. while my husband was driving. I suddenly became nauseated. I frequently got car sick, but that time it felt different. I told my mother that I had a strong suspicion that I may be pregnant. I quickly put that thought out of my mind, because after my first pregnancy, my doctor had informed me that I would likely not be able to get pregnant again. I had to undergo several fertility treatments in my first pregnancy after battling PCOS, so my doctor did not think it would be likely at all without fertility treatments again. Although I had always dreamed of having a baby girl as well, the cost of the fertility treatments were extremely high and my husband and I were just blessed to have a healthy baby boy. I couldn't be pregnant but I prayed that I was. Well much to my surprise, I was in fact pregnant and we were elated that God had answered our prayers.

At the time, I was working in one of the leading construction companies in Michigan, as a project engineer. Back then, the field was almost all male, but I had successfully navigated the ranks in the industry since I was 21 years old. I had become pretty comfortable with being the minority as a Black female in construction, although small hiccups along the way served as reminders that I was the minority. When I found out that I was pregnant, my employer was not exactly excited nor supportive. I ended up resigning from the job as it was no longer a good fit for me and my family.

About six months into the pregnancy, it was January and it had just snowed outside. I bundled up in my winter coat, scarf, hat, and gloves because Detroit winters were always freezing cold. I headed to the Detroit Medical Center for my routine prenatal check-up. My doctor was one of the few Black OBGYNs at the time in the Detroit area and his office stayed pretty busy. When he finally came into my room, he asked me the typical questions: if I had any contractions, cramping, leaking of fluid, bleeding, etc. I told him that I felt great and had no issues. I did have some occasional cramping, but nothing that I was concerned about. He decided it would be best if he checked my cervix just in case anyways. After I sat up, he explained to me that I was 2 centimeters dilated, in early labor, and I needed to go to the hospital immediately. We lived about 10–12 minutes from the medical center so I rushed home. I called my husband,

Melvin, and told him that I was in early labor and needed to go to Hutzel Hospital. He came home from work and we went to the hospital.

Luckily I had not dilated any further but when I was put onto the monitor, we realized that there were several contractions that were being picked up but I was not feeling. I was admitted for observation overnight. It wasn't exactly the most comfortable night, as they had my bed tilted with my head down toward the ground and my legs toward the ceiling. They told me this was a preventative measure to keep my baby girl in. Whatever it took to keep me pregnant, I was willing to do. I was discharged the next day with a fetal monitor that hooked up to our phone. The office could check in on my contractions every day without me having to be in the hospital. This was so different from my first pregnancy where my son refused to come out even past the due date, requiring them to induce me. Ironically, my second child can't wait to come out and see the world and she wasn't even full term yet. I was on bed rest the remaining months of my pregnancy. When I finally got to full term, Tamika had the nerve to be breech. I knew from that moment that my baby girl was going to make her own path. I ended up having to have a Cesarean section since Tamika was comfortable in the position that she wanted to be in and it was not head down, nor conducive to a vaginal delivery!

My husband and I knew she was going to be a force to reckon with. She was impatient since she was in my womb. This continued on throughout life and has fueled her self-starter, ambitious personality. She wanted to do everything and do it well. Tamika has always been a perfectionist and a very hardworking student (even in pre-school) while being involved with every extracurricular activity possible. Bedtime was always difficult in the Cross household because Tamika would never go to sleep. She was always awake thinking or planning and had an extreme fear of missing out.

I honestly think that sometimes she was planning out her next business venture because we saw the spark of her entrepreneurial spirit; from selling items in her room, to lemonade stands, to selling pens, braiding hair, doing nails... the list goes on. Raising a young, kindhearted girl with so much energy, determination, and wit taught us a lot about parenting with several challenges along the way. I remember my husband reading to Tamika every night and trying to skip a few pages here and there to hurry to the end. Even before she could read, she had the books memorized and would explain that he is skipping parts of the story and make him start over. There was never a dull moment in raising her. It has been amazing to see our baby grow into a beautiful, successful woman that overcomes every obstacle thrown her way.

Introduction

"Ok. Who is rounding on our antepartum unit this week?" Dr. Whitty asked while walking into the resident lounge. Dr. Whitty was the director of obstetrical services at the county hospital I was working at. She is a maternal fetal medicine (MFM) physician, often referred to as a high-risk pregnancy specialist. Although she was relatively new to the program, I knew Dr. Whitty from medical school when I was at Meharry Medical College in Nashville, Tennessee. She and I had a lot in common, including her living in Detroit for quite some time as she worked in the Detroit Medical Center and was a faculty member at Wayne State University medical school. She had relocated to Houston just two years before I did and I was excited to be able to work alongside her intimately. Her resume is impressive and she is a legend in the field of obstetrics in Detroit. She has published research papers, written chapters in well-known medical textbooks, and was triple boarded in obstetrics and gynecology, maternal fetal medicine, and critical care medicine. She was a walking encyclopedia. Although a native of New York, having her here in Houston with me felt like I had a piece of home here. Someone I could connect with, look up to, and learn a great deal from.

Every week, we had a different attending round on the service with us. For the antepartum team, these were our high-risk obstetrical patients meaning these women had medical problems that required hospitalization, were still pregnant, and we did our best to keep them that way as long as possible. For this service, we always had a second-year resident who rounded on the patients, meaning we interviewed and examined them each morning, wrote a note, and gave report to the MFM doctor on service that week. The second-year resident was responsible for managing their care throughout their hospital stay with the help of their chief resident and the attending physician. I was the resident on service that month.

"It's me, Dr. Whitty! I will be the resident rounding with you this week." I reported as I walked toward the door to join her. We were just finishing the morning report which is when the night team of doctors would give their report on the patients admitted to the hospital to the day time medical team. This transition typically took place at 7 AM and 5:30 PM every day. It consisted of each resident going to the front of the room, giving a formal check out on each patient on why the patient was there, how they did overnight, and what the plan was moving forward. This was also a time where attendings taught on various topics. I found these meetings to be extremely helpful because it stuck better when you learned about different medical topics and could attach it to a real life clinical scenario. I enjoyed learning this way much more than sitting in a library for hours with no clinical reference. Attending physicians would ask medical students and residents questions they expected them to know, and when they didn't, they were expected to go look it up. Although it may sound like a breeze, most residents and medical students can tell you that it can be quite stressful. It's great practice at presenting patients formally in a succinct matter which is a required skill for the rest of your career as a doctor.

After Dr. Whitty and I ran the patient list of the antepartum unit and she knew who was there and what our general plan was for each patient, we headed out to the hallway to start seeing the patients together. Sometimes, we only had a couple patients on this service, but most times, we had a full census. Working at the county hospital, we had very high-risk obstetrical patients with heart disease, preeclampsia, diabetes, kidney disease, and many of them had little to no prenatal care. Our job was so important because for many of these uninsured women, that was the first and possibly the last time they saw a doctor during their pregnancy before coming back in when they go into spontaneous labor. For that reason, we had to comb through their medical records with a fine tooth comb, run various labs, and ask more detailed questions to ensure we were providing the best medical care we can for our patients and their unborn child. Rounds took a very long time.

"Ms. Garcia is a nineteen-year-old G1P0 at 22 weeks gestation with no prenatal care who presented with pyelonephritis. She is now hospital day number two. She reports feeling somewhat better with the IV antibiotics, but still has severe back pain. Her TMax overnight was 101.4 degrees at 3 AM. Her pulse is a little elevated at 115, but her blood pressure has remained normotensive throughout the night. On exam, she has costovertebral angle tenderness bilaterally but more pronounced on the right side. Her white blood count is continuing to trend upward. She had an MFM ultrasound yesterday that showed that the baby is doing well and growing appropriately," I reported, as we were outside Ms. Garcia's room. In essence, this patient had a severe kidney infection that was not improving with our standard IV antibiotic regimen. We needed to do something different for her.

"So what do you want to do for her, Dr. Cross?" Dr. Whitty questioned.

"Well, I want to get imaging of her kidneys. She is now on her second day of IV antibiotics and she is not clinically improving. We need to rule out an abscess or some other etiology," I stated.

"Bingo! Put the order in stat. Be sure to tell the radiology department that I don't want her off the unit for too long. She looks pretty ill, and these patients can turn the corner quickly," she demanded.

"Yes ma'am," I responded as I went to the nearest computer station to put the order in while she was heading to the next patient's room without me. The radiology department was on the first floor, so in order to get any imaging done, our patients had to go downstairs from the second floor where the majority of them were on. In some instances, they would come to the patient and perform the imaging in the room, but these images never came out as clear and it was limited more to portable X-ray machines or certain bedside ultrasounds. As soon as I got off the phone with the radiology department, I joined Dr. Whitty to finish rounding on the other patients.

An hour and a half went by and we had finished rounding on all the patients. I stepped back into the resident lounge to put some more orders in and follow up on pending lab results that were not back earlier when Dr. Whitty and I rounded. My phone rang.

"Hi it's Dr. Cross, with OB," I answered the phone. As the second-year resident, not only did we care for antepartum obstetrical patients, we also performed repeat Cesarean sections, took gynecology consults on the floor and in the emergency room, and of course helped wherever else our chief resident needed us to.

"Hey it's Jackie on 2B. We have a patient in 204 who is nauseous, can she get some medicine for her nausea, please?" the nurse requested.

"Sure, I will have my intern come evaluate the patient and put in the necessary orders," I replied and got off the phone. I still had more charts to get through.

Beep! Beep! My pager was going off with the loud piercing noise. The sound being so annoying and loud is great when you're in the middle of surgery or a loud emergency room, but when it's right next to you in a quiet lounge, that thing can startle you! I looked at the green screen and saw the number I knew all too well—the emergency room. I called the number back and I was correct, it was the emergency room resident who had a consult for me downstairs. A patient who was 19 weeks pregnant and could not stop vomiting and showed clinical signs of dehydration. In most hospitals, pregnant women under 20 weeks are seen in the emergency room, while pregnant women above 20 weeks are automatically seen upstairs on our floor in the OB ED, also known as the Obstetrical Emergency Department. Dr. Whitty walked into the lounge to check if I was done with the charts. I was finishing up on the phone with the ER doctor.

"New consult downstairs?" she asked.

"Yep, 19 weeks, sounds like hyperemesis gravidarum. I will call you after I see her." I said. It was common practice for the resident to see the patient first, gather the information and perform the exam, then call the attending to present the patient. This is then followed by the attending coming to see the patient with you. Sometimes, in essence of time, our attending would just come down with us. This was one of those times.

"I'll just come downstairs with you to see her. Sounds like she is going to need to be admitted for IV hydration at the very least," Dr. Whitty suggested.

We headed downstairs and took a back hallway to get to the ER that was for staff only. It was a shortcut and although I had only been a resident there for a few months, I knew the hospital like the back of my hand. As a resident, we spend more time in the hospital than we do at our own homes. Taking the shortcut route, we had to pass by the radiology suite. Our patient Ms. Garcia was still downstairs.

"Let's go check on Ms. Garcia really quick since we are down here. Pyelonephritis patients get really sick really fast in pregnancy and she didn't look too well earlier. Let's just make sure she is ok," Dr. Whitty suggested. I agreed. It can't hurt to check in on our patient. Instead of making a left to the ER, we turned right and went toward the radiology suite. We found our patient pretty easily and she was next to get her kidney ultrasound. She looked up at us with a faint smile.

"Hey Ms. Garcia. We just wanted to check on you and see how you were feeling." Dr. Whitty turned to the radiology technician, "We are the doctors taking care of her, but we just wanted to check on her since her pulse was mildly elevated earlier."

The radiology technician smiled at us. "No problem. She seems ok, but she hasn't said much to me. We just wheeled her back here."

She was still hooked up to the monitor that read her pulse and blood pressure. Her pulse was at 160 beats per minute. This was significantly higher than before and what we had feared. Her blood pressure cycled and the reading said 96/61. This was not good. Her blood pressure was dropping and pulse was rising; she had a known source of infection. Our patient was going into septic shock. She appeared extremely drowsy.

"Ms. Garcia, are you feeling ok?" I questioned. She looked at me with her eyes barely open and was obviously too weak to respond. I turned to Dr. Whitty, "I think we need to call a rapid response!"

"I agree!" she declared. The radiology technician looked frazzled. I went over behind the desk and picked up the phone to call the rapid response that would then echo on the P.A. system of the entire hospital. This would bring more hands on deck including skilled nurses, other physicians, and ancillary staff to assist in an emergency. We were in the middle of the radiology suite. Ms. Garcia had an IV but she needed an additional IV and more fluids to help bring her blood pressure up. An intensive care unit (ICU) nurse was the first to arrive with a crash cart that had supplies that we would need to support the patient. She ran into the suite with her rolling cart coming to an abrupt halt.

"Thanks for coming! I'm Dr. Cross and this Dr. Whitty, we are the OB physicians taking care of her. This patient is 22 weeks pregnant with pyelonephritis and going into septic shock. We need two large bore IVs STAT. What fluids do you have in your cart?" I asked. She gave me a blank stare.

"Why did you call a rapid response on this patient? She isn't unresponsive. She looks fine." She challenged. *Really*?! I was taken aback. The patient was not unresponsive and we wanted to keep it that way, she was entering septic shock and needed emergent fluid resuscitation.

"We need two large bore IVs stat!" Dr. Whitty interjected. The nurse gave her a blank stare as well.

At that point the other members of the rapid response team arrived including the ICU attending, Dr. Green and his resident. After giving a brief one-line synopsis of what was going on to Dr. Green, he turned to the ICU nurse.

"Why haven't you put in two large bore IVs yet? It was ordered stat." He glanced over at the patient's vital signs again. "She is in septic shock and needs fluid resuscitation immediately!"

"Yes, doctor! Right away!" the nurse said hurriedly while flinging open the drawers to the crash cart and grabbing the supplies needed. She continued to ignore both Dr. Whitty and me during the remainder of the time she was there as if we did not exist.

After stabilizing the patient, and the rapid response team started to dissipate, Dr. Green stepped outside in the hallway with Dr. Whitty, me, his resident, and the charge nurse. He was a middle-aged white male who stood about six feet tall. He had the same white coat that Dr. Whitty and I had on as we all worked for the same academic institution. His ID badge was clasped from his lapel as was ours and it had the same letters following his last name, M.D. His face was bright red.

"You know I appreciate you both calling us to help out. So often we are called too late in the process so I am glad you both intervened quickly. We will take her to our ICU to continue to stabilize her and we would appreciate you all following her as well, to make recommendations for the pregnancy," he stated.

Our hospital had a closed ICU which means when your patient goes to the ICU, typically, they are managing the patient primarily. This is to avoid "too many cooks in the kitchen" and to help reduce the amount of physicians making decisions on one patient. Although it was a closed unit, whenever there was a pregnant patient, they wanted us to follow along to make recommendations from a pregnancy standpoint as that was not their field. We didn't mind that approach, after all, she was our patient and we had been caring for and her unborn baby for the past couple days. He paused with a long sigh. "I also want to apologize for what happened in there. Trisha is one of our best ICU nurses and I've never seen her behave that way toward a physician. I am embarrassed."

"We appreciate that, Dr. Green." Dr. Whitty said calmly. *That's it? Nothing more?* I was outraged and my blood was boiling inside. Dr. Whitty was calm. There she stood, a triple-boarded physician trained in critical care medicine, with an extensive nursing background prior to becoming a physician, author of chapters of the top medical textbooks, who is also the director of our entire unit and sat as the head on multiple hospital committees, and was overlooked as a physician by Trisha. Now I forgot to mention that Dr. Whitty is a Black female physician who was nearing retirement.

She has a petite frame that she kept in shape with weekly body pump classes and a healthy diet. She has golden brown naturally curly hair, always stylish, and is the definition of goals. I couldn't believe this was happening before my eyes.

"I am going to report her. This is inexcusable and could have cost the patient her life and her little one!" the charge nurse interrupted. There was really nothing to say at that point. The only person I had wanted to say something to was the ICU nurse that completely ignored us. But what was that going to accomplish? Although this wasn't the first time I was passed over, looked over, disrespected, mistaken for anything else but the doctor, I had never seen it happen to my attending—my boss—the person who I looked up to.

Because of the many times it happened to minority physicians, we soon became desensitized to it. The excuses of our colleagues were always about how we were dressed, or how young we looked, or that they simply did not know who we were. What was the excuse this time? Both of us dressed in long white coats over our scrubs, with badges that said Medical Doctor. She was well known around the hospital as she sat on several committees and was one of the directors there. I was 26 years old, but Dr. Whitty, a seasoned physician, was also ignored. On top of it all, we announced who we were the second the ICU nurse walked into the room so there were no mistakes. She wasn't hard of hearing, she wasn't confused about who we were, or where we were from. She simply did not want to take orders from the two Black female doctors.

Dr. Whitty and I talked for a while after this incident. I was in disbelief. I needed her support in that moment when I was filled with emotion. I knew how much I had been questioned over my first two years as a doctor, but I didn't realize that even after forty plus years into my career like Dr. Whitty, I would still be facing the same ugly truth. Five percent of all physicians are Black. Two percent of all physicians are Black women. We know that we are unicorns and people are surprised to see that we exist. I just hate that when we show up, dress the part, and introduce ourselves accordingly, that we are still not treated with the same dignity and respect as our White or male counterparts. I always had hope that there was a light at the end of the tunnel, that after residency I wouldn't continue to face this ugly truth. Standing there next to a well-known, accomplished, triple-boarded Black female physician, facing the same discrimination as me, I knew this would be a long uphill battle.

Defeated, I returned to the resident physician lounge where I was met by two other residents. I couldn't hide my frustration at this point. I told them what had just happened and how I was still in disbelief. Their response was unforgettable.

"That's crazy that happened to you! I'm sure it's not because you're Black though. You do look kind of young to be a doctor, Tamika!" one laughed.

"What about Dr. Whitty? Does she look like a doctor?" I asked. Silence.

What's even more difficult than navigating the tumultuous journey of becoming a doctor, and having your credentials questioned every single place you go, is having colleagues who do not understand your plight or even attempt to understand. It may sound like us "complaining" or "playing the race card" or not accepting that it is a "big misunderstanding", but until one walks the hospital wards in our shoes, they cannot fathom how different our experience truly is. Being interrupted during patient interviews by family members or patients who continue to ask "When is the doctor coming by?", or being handed a food tray or a bedpan full of urine or stool when you walk into your patient's room, being asked if you graduated from high school, or having a patient whose baby you just delivered last night tell their spouse "hold on baby, my nurse is in here", or even plainly being told "I don't want a Black doctor" is an added layer to an already stressful, time consuming, career. Excuses such as: you look young, they don't know you, it was just a mistake... these can only last so long. Many people seem to have this prototype of what they expect to see when their doctor walks into the room, but my question is *what does a doctor look like?*

Part I

The Egg (Pre-college)

CHAPTER 1

Brainwash Your Perm

"I need to see my own beauty and to continue to be reminded that I am enough, that I am worthy of love without effort, that I am beautiful, that the texture of my hair and that the shape of my curves, the size of my lips, the color of my skin, and the feelings that I have are all worthy and okay."

–Tracee Ellis Ross

"Did you have a good day, TT?" my mom questioned while driving my brother and me home from daycare. TT was a nickname that I hold near and dear to my heart. Even to this day, my family still calls me TT, including my two adorable nephews.

"Yes, we had fun, Mommy. We learned a new song, played outside for extra time because we were good and got to paint with our fingers!" I exclaimed.

"Well that sounds like a fun day to me," my mom replied.

"Juliana could not play with Vicki and me today, so she played with some of the boys, but she did not look like she had as much fun as us!"

Perplexed, my mom asked, "Well how come she could not play with you two? Did she get in trouble?"

"No. Her mommy and daddy said she can't play with Black kids," I responded.

That scenario did not really make sense to me at the time nor did it set in until a few years later. But my older brother, Melvin, was old enough to understand back then. I'm not sure if that was his first time experiencing racism, but it surely was mine. Being too young to understand, I was more frustrated with losing my "friend" than I was over the "reason why". We had been playing together for a few weeks since she came to the school, and I always had been really nice to Juliana. *Why did she not want to be my friend anymore?* As clueless as I was at the time, this situation has remained engraved in my memory.

I loved my childhood daycare, Bright Horizons. Not only did it feel like a family environment, I enjoyed interacting with other kids my age. Many of my cousins that were the same age as me lived in other states and I only got a chance to see them for special holidays and summers. Bright Horizons was a warm and friendly home for both my brother me and we attended there for years. My mom even started working part time there and was considering becoming an owner of the daycare. We learned, we played, we sang, and we danced. I always had an enjoyable experience there.

Juliana was a nice girl. She was the same age as my friends and me so we always played together. One day, she came to school with a different intention. She came right up to me and my friend Vicki and said, "My parents said I cannot play with you two anymore because you are Black!" Vicki and I exchanged confused faces and continued playing with our other friends for the rest of the day. Not fully understanding this moment to be my first exposure to racism at age four, I certainly didn't understand that it would not be my last.

At the time, we were living on the west side of Detroit, Michigan and many of the people around me looked like me. It wasn't until I started interacting with kids from different backgrounds that I realized the major differences. Having always been a busybody, in particular, dancing every time I heard music (even if the music was just in my head) my parents knew that I loved to dance. My parents enrolled me in dance class at a young age, and from there, a deep love and appreciation grew for the art. Dance was easily one of my first loves. I enjoyed all types of dance; from ballet, to tap, to modern, to jazz. Tap dance was always my favorite as a child, and I was excited every time we had a tap routine for our recitals because I knew that we were going to be focusing more time on it.

Although we lived in Detroit at the time, my first dance school was in a suburb, Royal Oak, Michigan. In the early 90's, the area was almost all White and lacked diversity, although one could argue it hasn't changed significantly even today. My dance school reflected the same demographic, with me being the only Black girl in my class and one of the few Black girls in the entire school.

Being in dance at such a young age, I wasn't keen on the many differences between my dance friends and me. For recitals, I remember being backstage with other dancers and the stage moms who helped get all of us "stage ready". This included helping us put on our costumes, getting our stage makeup applied, and making sure our hair was pulled nice and neat into a high bun. One of my earliest memories of our dance recitals was that the "preferred makeup" shades looking different on my skin tone. Bright blue eye shadow and red lips look very different on my melanin-rich skin and full lips than my white counterparts regardless of how fair skinned I appear.

"Tamika, get over here so I can touch up your hair!" My mom demanded while I was running around with my classmates backstage. We had spent all night in the kitchen straightening my hair with a hot comb. I absolutely hated getting my hair pressed. I loved how it looked in the end, but I always cringed when the hot comb came near my edges, or the hot steam would come close to my face. Even worse was when she had to press the hair near my ears. She always had me grab the top of my ears and fold them down to help protect them from being burned. Quite honestly, the hot sizzle from melting Blue Magic grease would pop on my skin and would be just as uncomfortable as if the actual metal touched my skin directly. I could be in the back of the house playing with Barbies in my bedroom and smell the aroma of burned hair and oils and I knew exactly what time it was. Our first hot comb was not electric. It was a metal comb on a wooden handle and we sat it on the oven burner to get hot. When the oils and old hair on the comb would heat up, the smell was unforgettable. I can always smell the aroma of burned hair and oils when I even think about walking into any Black hair salon to this day.

Despite spending all night straightening my hair for my dance recital and slicking my edges down with Murray's beeswax, after running around with my friends, my naturally curly and coarse hair would begin to curl up around the edges. Since I was the only Black girl in my dance class, and the only one with tightly coiled hair, no one else had this issue. I knew I wasn't supposed to be running around "sweating my hair out" before going on stage, but I was four years old and it was hard to resist. Since it took a little bit of extra work to get my thick, natural, curly hair slicked up in a high bun on top of my head, this was not a task that could be achieved in a few minutes before it was our turn on stage. My mom frequently volunteered as a stage mom to help us get ready. But I knew secretly, she was the only mom that knew what it took to get my hair brushed, slicked, and pulled into the required high bun, especially in the event of me messing it up like I just had. She also always had my own makeup in my bag for sanitary purposes as well as being able to choose a slightly different shade that would look more pleasant on my skin tone.

Although subtle, and few, these small differences were observed at a young age when I started to shift in recognizing my identity as a little Black girl. I don't recall feeling any negative or ill feelings on being different than my peers in this setting, nor do I recall any teasing or remarks about my skin color or hair. I actually enjoyed standing out a little bit, as my family always had an easy time spotting me on stage for pictures and videos! As I grew older, more of the subtle differences became more prevalent, and I appreciated a transition to a new dance school that had more diversity in dancers, body types, themes, and music. I loved to dance and would be happy dancing anywhere, but I would be lying if I said there wasn't an unexplainable level of comfort in being around girls who did look like me, had similar backgrounds as me, used similar hair products and makeup tones and shades as me.

Over the years, I realized that I would have many situations of feeling "different" because of my race. I was a little Black girl from Detroit, now living in the suburbs, who danced at an all White dance school, played tennis, and was on the swim team. Not exactly the set up to be around other people who looked like me. It was all I came to know so it did not bother me to be around people who did not look like me at that time.

It wasn't until I became old enough to start liking boys, listening to my own music, and visiting friends' houses, that I realized major differences. Let me emphasize, MAJOR DIFFERENCES. I did not want to listen to the newest Hansen hit on replay. I wanted to listen to the music my family listened to at home and family gatherings, and it certainly was not that. When we put up posters of the cutest celebrity crushes, my friends and I did not ever seem to agree. I wasn't exactly "checking for" the white teen boy groups at the time. I was more into the artists who were typically found in *Word Up!* magazines, and trust me when I say none of my friends owned or probably even heard of this magazine back then!

If you haven't guessed it by now, two of my best friends growing up were White. We didn't seem to let race define our friendship despite what society told us. But I would be lying if I said that it did not come up on a regular basis. I had to have my hair "prepped" for swimming and summers. Meaning I needed my cornrows in because it was the easiest way to manage my thick unruly hair after getting it wet. And if I went swimming without a swimming cap like my friends did, I knew that I would not hear the end of it when I got home. There were even times that I found myself telling my friends I couldn't play that day because I needed to get my hair done.

Wash day was just that; a whole day's worth of work. It would not consist of me washing my hair in the shower and letting it air dry while I go out to play. We had to wash, condition, detangle, deep condition, blow dry, and then... a few several hours later, we were ready to BEGIN the hairstyle of choice. When I was old enough to start getting "perms", I cannot even begin to explain the frustration of trying to explain why I couldn't scratch my head for the few days leading up to my appointment.

To all my possibly uninformed readers, a permanent (commonly referred to as a "perm") was a highly potent chemical that people (mainly Black women) put on their hair to make it straight. It has to sit on your hair long enough to change the chemical properties and break down and restructure the protein bonds in the hair follicles. This restructuring would cause the hair to not curl up and get frizzy when wet, and just stay bone straight (sorry for the super nerdy description. Y'all know I have a science background, so let me live). It was a creamy white substance that Black women relied on to keep their hair "manageable" to societal standards; straight, silky, smooth, no kinks, no curls, no waves. The exact opposite of how our hair naturally grew out of our scalp. Due to its appearance and Black women's dependence on it, it coined the nickname, "creamy crack" although that may not sound politically correct in this day and age.

I explained to my friends that the chemicals made my hair straight and if I scratched my scalp or combed my hair too much on "perm day" I would end up with bad chemical burns and scabs all over my head. I knew this all too well from experience.

"Now Tamika, be sure to tell me when you start feeling burning on your scalp and I will rinse it out," my hairdresser Chuck would remind me every time. I knew the routine of getting a perm all too well and quite honestly didn't need the reminder.

"Ok!" I confidently said. I always knew "the longer, the better." I never told him it was burning as soon as the burning would start. The one time I did that, he rinsed it out immediately and the perm did not "take" well. This meant that my hair wasn't as straight and was not left on long enough to see the desired effects. It always felt like a waste of time, because I had to wait another 6 to 8 weeks to try again. So I adopted a policy like many other Black girls and women. I wanted my hair to be silky smooth after my perm, so a little burning was considered "part of the process". I would try to hold out until it was burning unbearably, then I would have him urgently rinse the chemical off my hair.

This dangerous, harsh chemical is potent enough to unclog drains, strip paint off wood, used in industrial cleaning, yet we were putting it on our scalp to straighten our hair. We did all of this because without a perm, our hair was considered "unprofessional and unkempt". While "natural hairstyles" may appear to be the latest fad these days, it was not always this way. Cornrows, locs, afros, twists and puffballs are even still frequently labeled as unprofessional in many schools and jobs. I never understood why other people had an opinion about the hair that grows out of OUR scalp. Even celebrities weren't exempt from the discrimination regarding their hair. Oprah Winfrey was told that her hair was too thick and was forced to get a perm that resulted in her going completely bald for quite a long time. We have constantly been told that our hair was undesirable in the natural styles. The brainwashing and self-hate mentality this process encompasses makes me sick to my stomach currently while thinking about it. We felt the need to conform that bad that we put ourselves through chemical burns even as a child. Ugh!

"Tamika, why do you put those chemicals in your hair? I just wash mine and let it dry and then it's straight. Maybe you should try that too," my friend Sally suggested. She just did not understand that without this perm, if I wet my hair and let it air dry, my hair would be a large, tangled, curly afro puff that would add at least another two to three hours to my hair routine. This whole hair ordeal may not seem like much now, but as a child with White friends who wanted to run outside and play, it was a big deal to me!

Confession. I went through my conformation phase too! When I finally started getting relaxers, I would be excited to go swimming without a shower cap. My hair would be bone straight and long like my friends and teammates and not a huge nappy Afro. This made me feel more like them and I enjoyed it. I was still supposed to wear my swim cap because my mom warned me that with the strong chemicals I had in my hair, I needed to be careful about getting chlorine in it everyday. She explained that over time, it could damage my hair and cause it to break off. Anytime my hair got wet in the pool, I was supposed to wash it using a special shampoo to get all of the chlorine out, condition it, rinse it out, then blow dry it. Even with a perm in my head, this routine would take hours so I, like any other kid, cut corners. With my mom working evenings at this time, my dad was bringing us home from swim practice, and supervising the bedtime routines. I definitely took advantage of that. I knew my dad was not going to pay attention to my hair routine like my mom did. I frequently would come home from practice and if my hair was wet, unbeknownst to my parents, I would just blow dry it and go to bed. Little did I know that years later, this sneaky, unhealthy hair routine would catch up to me and result in major hair breakage from the retained chemicals and require a haircut that I wouldn't like. There I was thinking I was "winning" when in actuality, I was setting myself up to lose major inches off my hair. Yikes!

Another area that I felt the need to "fit in" was with girl talk. I literally used to lie about having crushes on the "hottest boys at the pool" (all of who were White) just to feel accepted. But in reality, I wasn't attracted to all of them. Now I did have my first crush on a White boy from my swim team. He was pretty popular and many of the other girls liked him too. My giggly obnoxious friends approached him one day to see if he liked me. His response was, "Tamika? She's Black..." as if that was an answer in itself. I remember feeling surprised but not defeated. I liked him, but that didn't crush me like one would expect. In my head, it seemed unrealistic anyways, so I got over it fast. Although I had bi-racial friends, and saw parents of different backgrounds who were together, I did not see that in kids my age at that time. Kids my age seemed to pretty much stick to dating people of their same race, so to me, a White boyfriend at that time felt unrealistic anyways.

One of my fondest childhood memories were our many family vacations. My mom worked for Northwest Airlines (which is now Delta Airlines) when I was younger. She had major perks being an airline employee and my brother and I loved flying first class sometimes and being able to go on vacation at least a couple times of year. My grandpa lived in Orlando, so the Disney experience was one that we frequented quite a bit. We basically flew for free, and my grandpa lived in driving distance from the parks. It was a win-win situation for us kids. Although my grandpa lived nearby, we often grabbed hotels that had kid friendly amenities that my brother Melvin and I enjoyed.

That one particular Disney trip, I was about 8 or 9 years old and Melvin was 11 years old. We hopped in a cab at the airport and headed to the hotel our parents had booked. We pulled up and I still remember the feeling of amazement. I was amazed at how large the resort was, and how fancy it seemed. It was a very upscale, Victorian style resort with tall cathedral ceilings. My brother and I couldn't wait to get out of the cab and check the hotel out. There were bellhops approaching cars and cabs as they pulled up. They would open the door and grab everyone's bags as the family would be escorted to the front desk to check into their hotel suite. Wow! I thought *if this is what royalty felt like, I dreamed of becoming royalty one day!* Our cab pulled up at the front door and waited a couple minutes that felt like forever to my eight-year-old self.

No one came to our cab.

"Alright. Everyone get out and grab your bags!" My dad ordered with a bit of annoyance in his tone. We hopped out the cab with haste! It was our spring break at school. Back home in Detroit, the weather was super cold. Now we were in Florida, and it was hot! We wanted to do what all kids would want to do with this climate change! We were ready to go swimming. My brother and I were already making a mental checklist of all the things we couldn't wait to do after we got to our room and changed into our summer clothes!

No one approached us to assist with our bags.

We grabbed our own bags and headed inside to check in. Everyone was being escorted to the front desk or being approached by staff to assist with whatever their needs were. My parents tried to flag someone down.

We were ignored.

My mom was seemingly getting frustrated and talking with my dad off to the side. My parents told us to go stand by the side door. It was a small area that was out of the entrance so we would not be in the way of arriving guests. My brother and I obeyed and re-focused our attention on the salamanders we saw running around by the bushes. We didn't have these in Michigan so we always had a good time spotting them in Florida because they were everywhere! I remember my nosey little self looking over to where my parents were at the front desk. *What was taking so long?* Every other hotel we had been to, we typically checked in pretty quickly, got our room keys, and we were on our way. More than an hour had passed. My dad occasionally came over to make sure we were ok.

"Melvin, are y'all ok?" he asked.

"Yea, we are good, dad!" Melvin replied.

I interjected, "Daddy what's taking so long? We want to go swimming then play putt-putt golf!" This was not unusual. Melvin being calm and collected, and me being impatient, anxious, and ready to jump into our next activity.

"We are working out some kinks right now. Stay here and don't move," Dad stated.

"Yes, sir," I grudgingly responded.

Another 45 minutes or so went by and honestly at that point, I didn't care about seeing any more stupid lizards. I was bored, sitting on a bench, when I should have been racing my brother in the pool by now! My parents walked over to us. We jumped up.

"Yay! Finally! What floor are we on? Can I hold one of the keys please?" I was super excited.

"Grab your bags. We are leaving." My dad informed us in a dry tone.

"But why—" I started to ask.

"Tamika, it's not a good time for questions. Grab your things like your father said and let's go," my mom said firmly.

I truly didn't understand what was going on. Why was everyone in such a bad mood now? Why were we leaving this super ritzy hotel? We finally had a chance to stay in this castle and now we have to leave. This was not fair. I had so many questions, but I knew better than to continue asking them at this time. My parents' body language kept me quiet even though my inquisitive mind was going 100 miles a minute.

We pulled up to another a hotel that was only a short cab ride away. It was nice as well, but it didn't have the same "royalty" vibe as the first hotel. Everyone was friendly, check-in was quick and we got to our room in under 20 minutes. The rest of our vacation was a blast. It wasn't explained to me what had happened for at least a few years. Apparently the staff continued to ignore my parents. After my dad insisted on speaking with someone, they were treated like second-class citizens. From condescending remarks, to lack of attentiveness, my parents had a very negative experience that was not new to them, but they certainly did not want us exposed to it at that time. They did not want to kill the positive energy of our trip which is why they were so adamant about me not discussing it further. Needless to say, we never visited that hotel again.

Several encounters took place throughout my childhood that stood out to me as "abnormal" but I was too young to have a full understanding until later. As I grew older and when my family and I would reminisce on various memories, I always learned more about those situations that my naïveté barred me from seeing as a child. Those situations each taught me a great deal about myself and aided in the discovery of my identity at a young age.

What was more frustrating than not being "White enough" to fit in with my White friends, was not being "Black enough" to make new Black friends. I cannot count how many times I was told by peers that I "talked White" for using proper grammar or pronouncing words differently than others. What did "talking White" even mean? I used to shrug it off in an unbothered fashion, but in actuality, it bothered me a lot. Having a fair skin complexion, I was always asked if I was mixed, as if this was maybe the justification for me "talking White". I don't know anyone who is not mixed to some degree, but at that age, it was basically asking were one of my parents non-Black. The simple answer is no; both of my parents identify as Black, as do I.

As I got older and started hanging around more friends that looked like me, I realized that things were different. From the music, to the latest dances, the fashion, and the slang. I mean, I didn't emerge from under a rock exactly, but there were vast differences that I noticed the second I entered my middle school. I enjoyed having friends with similar backgrounds as me and similar taste in music, fashion, and boys! I continued to get the occasional "you talk White" remarks, but I soon learned to ignore them even at that age, I didn't fully grasp what that even meant.

There was a pivotal turning point in my childhood when I decided that I was going to stop trying to be someone who I wasn't. I was just going to be me. I was not a Backstreet

Boys aficionado and also never wanted to listen to "Mmm Bop" ever again! I was the little Black girl, with super fair skin who got horrible sunburn in the summer, had kinky hair when it gets wet, swam competitively, played tennis, was attracted to Black boys, talked with proper grammar, loved school, and enjoyed hip hop music and dance. Soon, I became comfortable with that narrative.

Fast forward to some years later. My racist neighbor, Jade, whose family had made it very clear they did not like Black people, called me a nigger one day after school. Our families never got along because of the racial tensions, harassment, them throwing a brick at my dog, their mother chasing my brother and me home with a minivan—the list goes on. We learned to co-exist—going to the same school, riding the same school bus, and we just did not speak. I was ok with that, as was she.

One day on the bus ride home, some kids were throwing stuff at her. I was not sure why or what had happened at school, but I did witness them picking on her on the bus. At that time, our school system was much more integrated and majority of the students were Black. She was the minority. She turned around to me and my friend, Blake who were seated together and lived on the same street. She shouted "This is why I hate you niggers!" We had absolutely nothing to do with the kids taunting her on the bus. "Jade, just wait until we get off this bus! You're going to regret ever saying that!" I reassured her. The school bus dropped us off at our routine stop.

As soon as the bus pulled off, I asked Jade, "So what was that you said to us on the bus?"

She shouted "Just leave me alone, niggers!" while stomping down the street. My other friend was arguing back and forth with her, but as a guy, he was not going to put his hands on her. Well, I was a girl and I did not care at that point. I knocked her down with my book bag and I engaged in my first fist fight. As soon as she caught a break, she got up and took off running down the street.

She yelled, "This isn't the end of this, Tamika!" It surely wasn't. At the moment, I realized something had changed inside of me. I remembered the many times racial slurs and inappropriate comments had been directed toward me and I didn't do anything about it. This was my first time retaliating and saying enough was enough, and I did not care about the consequences—or so I thought. It did result in me getting called to the principal's office the next day (since this occurred at the "school bus stop") and my parents were informed. My mom already knew about the story at that point. I told her as soon as she got home from work that day. That was in part because our parents had always told them to inform them of the altercations we had with their family. The other reason was because the police station had called later that afternoon stating that she had filed a police report. The telephone rang.

"Hello?" I answered cautiously. We had just gotten a caller ID device and we could see who was calling. It read:

Lathrup Village Police Station. I almost shit my pants. *Was I going to jail?*

"Hello, is Mrs. Cross home?" the officer inquired. I knew I wasn't supposed to tell anyone when my parents weren't home, but he was a police officer so I answered honestly.

"No, sir. She is not home yet." I stuttered quietly.

"Well when she comes home, you and her need to come up to the police station. Your classmate Jade is here with her mother," he stated.

"Ok. I will tell her. Thanks!" I said in the nicest voice. I was terrified. I had never been in any serious trouble before. *Was I going to be arrested?* I did throw the first punch but she called me a nigger first. I prayed they would be understanding. *After all, I was a straight A honor student. This was just a "kid fight".* I immediately thought of the episodes of Cops my brother and I watched at night when we were supposed to be sleep. Some of those police officers were beating Black people's ass! *Were they going to beat me like that? Will I ever become a doctor if my record shows that I was locked up at the age of 12?* I was terrified.

When my mom came home, we headed up to the police station together. She wasn't happy but she also didn't reprimand me either. I didn't know what was about to happen. I know one thing, and that was that my mother was over this tension between our two families. This racial tension between Jade's family and ours was at least six years old. We pulled up at the police station and my palms were sweaty. I was seconds away from crying.

"Mommy, are they going to put me in jail? Are they going to beat me like on TV? What's going to happen? I'm sorry! I promise I won't do it ever again." I was on the brink of tears. I didn't realize how afraid I truly was until we parked in the parking lot.

"Baby, I'm here with you. None of that is going to happen. Get out the car. Everything will be ok," she reassured me.

We walked into the police station. Before we could open the front door, I saw Jade and her mother sitting off to the side. My mom looked at me.

"Now don't you say anything to them, you hear me?" she stated.

"Yes ma'am!" I agreed.

My mom knew how much I couldn't stand her and she knew that if she said something racist to me, that there was a chance I would react negatively again. We were at the police station because of years of pent up anger and frustration toward her, so she knew what I was capable of at that point. Her warning was warranted, and I obliged.

The police officer was sitting behind a desk and much to my surprise, he was a middle-aged Black man. He ran through the events that had taken place earlier that day and allowed each of us to speak during our turn. When asked if I had initiated the physical fight, I didn't hold back. I told him why I did and that she had called me a nigger twice; on the bus and off the bus. I also told him I had witnesses to prove it. He raised his eyebrow when the word nigger rolled of my tongue. He looked over his glasses at her and her mother.

"Jade, did you say that?" he questioned.

"Yes I did, because all of them were teasing me on the bus and throwing things at me," she defended. "They always act like that. They pick on me because I am not Black. They are the bullies, not me!"

After I explained that I was not a part of the group who was picking on her, she cut me off, "Yes you were! All you people do is pick on people who aren't Black! If you ask me, you're the racists!"

Offended by her phrase, the officer questioned, "All what people?"

Her mom cut in, "All you niggers! You're picking her side because you're a nigger too!"

The officer chuckled. This wasn't the type of chuckle someone uses when something actually is funny. This was the chuckle that had an undertone of "you better watch yourself." This led to a lobby of shouting racial slurs from Jade and her mother and also lucky for me, the officer tore up the police report. He asked them to leave and they continued on. He signaled for my mother and me to leave the station. We didn't hesitate and jetted out of there. When we got in the car, I let out a sigh of relief and a hearty laugh. My mom shot me a side eye.

"I understand why you did what you did today, Tamika, and I cannot say that I would have reacted differently. I know you and your brother are sick of them. Your father and I are sick of that family too. But at the end of the day, only you can control your actions. That situation could have led to a much worse outcome. I just want you to be safe, Tamika. Your father and I aren't always going to be there to protect you so I need you to make wise decisions. One wrong move in the wrong place at the wrong time can land you irreversible circumstances, especially being Black. You and your brother are to ignore her and her family from now on," she explained.

Although I hated getting lectured, I knew it was coming. I didn't truly appreciate the value in these words spoken to me until a much later date, but I knew to ignore them from that day forward. A part of me was still proud of myself—proud that I stood my ground and defended myself. I knew that Jade would think twice about calling me a nigger ever again.

My childhood memories are fond. I have no regrets about where I was from, where I lived or moved to, who I befriended, etc. Childhood definitely shapes us in our adult lives. Insecurities, fears, and hobbies can stem from these earliest memories. They shape how we view the world and most importantly how we view ourselves.

> ***Affirmation to recite:*** *I am unique by design. I am beautifully and wonderfully made. I am enough.*
>
> ***Question:*** *When have you, past or present, conformed? Why did you feel the need to? Do you still feel the need to conform? Why or why not?*

CHAPTER 2

You are talented. You are gifted.

"I never cut class. I loved getting As. I liked being smart. I liked being on time. I thought being smart is cooler than anything in the world."

—Michelle Obama

My parents were adamant about Melvin and me knowing how to swim. They didn't care about us competing or joining a team, but they wanted us to at least be able to save ourselves. In order to achieve that, our parents put us in swim classes at the YMCA starting at the youngest age they would allow. The swim classes at the YMCA were pretty small and only had about four or five kids per group. With Melvin and me being only a couple years apart in age, we were able to be in the same class, although our skill level was nowhere near equal.

I look up to my big brother so much, and have always wanted to be around him, especially as a kid. I honestly think being around him was what gave me the drive to do things "ahead of my time". When I saw him reading, I wanted to learn to read. When I saw him riding a bike without training wheels, I wanted to ride without training wheels. I'm that way today. I like to surround myself with people who push me to be better or can teach me something new or show me how to do something different. Some call this characteristic in me "competitive", but in actuality, it's just my drive to be better. Ok, maybe I am a little competitive, but in a healthy way! I like group boot camps better than one-on-one training because when everyone around me is still running laps or holding their plank, it makes me hold out longer. I think that's natural, right? If I am by myself, when I feel that burn, I drop to the floor panting. Ha!

The way the YMCA was set up was there was a huge glass window where spectators (parents and family), could sit behind and watch their children in swim class. My parents would always sit on the first bleacher in front of the glass. I remember often waving to them in the middle of class rather than paying attention sometimes. I hated sitting for the long instructional talks—let's just jump in and do it! This has always been my personality, and my friends and family would agree that nothing has changed about me in that regard.

On this particular day, we learned how to swim across the width of the pool in the deep end using a kickboard. I was about four years old, and Melvin was six. We had already graduated from wearing life vests and arm floating devices.

We held onto the blue foam kickboard that floated in the water and kicked our legs fast to propel our bodies forward. It was fun! Our teacher made sure to tell us to keep our legs stiff and straight and make small fast kicks. This helped with speed and was a mini introduction to proper form. After a few rounds, I had the hang of it. I was ready to swim without the board. Unfortunately, our teacher only allowed the older kids in the group to swim with no kickboard because they had been practicing for the past few weeks. He hadn't shown us how to do it yet. No fair! How hard could it be? If Melvin could do it, I could too! At the end of the class, we always gathered on the deck right next to the pool and discussed a few things we had learned. At the end of the huddle, we had to go to the opposite side of the pool where all of our flip flops were before heading into the locker room. This meant we had to walk all the way around the pool to get to the other side. Jared, our teacher, looked at Melvin and the other older kid in the group.

"You two can swim to the other side without kickboards if you want! Remember after you jump in, start kicking your legs like I taught you using your arms too!" They were so excited. They both jumped in and started swimming.

"I want to swim across too, Jared! I know I'm young but I promise I can do it too!" I whined.

"Not this time, Tamika. You're not ready yet, but you will be in no time!" Jared assured me. How was I not ready? Melvin and I swam outside of the YMCA recreationally all the time and I could do just about what he could. I knew how to jump in, tread water, and I'm sure I could swim without a stupid kickboard! The other kids started walking to the other side of the pool. As soon as Jared turned his back, I did what most kids with my stubborn ways and overly confident attitude would do. I jumped in.

I recall going deeper and deeper, still right next to the side of the pool, yet not using that to pull myself up. I opened my eyes under water and stared at the tile wall as my body went deeper and deeper. *How do I come back to the surface and start kicking again?* This wasn't a good time to realize that Jared was right and I didn't know how to come back up as we hadn't practiced it much in my age group. Apparently, my mom who was watching intently from behind the glass with my father was banging on the glass so hard she was surprised it didn't break. She was trying to get Jared's attention to let him know that I was under water. Once Jared caught wind of what my parents were trying to convey through the glass, he instantly jumped in and pulled me out the water.

Allegedly, I looked unbothered. No tears. Not scared. Just normal. I guess everyone expected the dramatic "drowning kid" scene from a movie with me coughing up water and crying and panting for my next breath. I wasn't anything like that. I didn't feel like I was drowning. I knew how to swim. I was under water, chilling, but just didn't know how to come back to the surface. If I was down there long enough, then maybe I would have had the exaggerated response everyone expected. He asked me why I jumped in when he specifically told me to walk around. My response was simple. "You let the two of them swim across, and I knew I could do it too!" I had an earful when I came out of swim class that day, while Melvin couldn't stop laughing.

"TT, what's wrong with you? Why did you jump in? You know you can't swim!" he teased.

"I can too! I just needed a little help!" I shouted. I didn't realize how much that floating kickboard was really holding me above water. Without it, I just kept sinking to the bottom. My parents were pissed, as they should have been, especially with the lack of remorse from my unbothered self who didn't realize how dangerous what I had just done really was. This has now become a laughing point in my family who tells this story to everyone. Most people who know me and hear this story aren't surprised one bit. My personality has always been the same. Never scared to try anything new, always wanted to be hands on, and always up for a challenge. I'm more of a "dive in and see what happens" kind of girl, sink or swim... literally!

At the daycare I attended, they began having kindergarten enrichment classes. I was too young as I was only four. However, I was a busybody and was always bored so they would let me sit in with the older kids who would come to the daycare after school for more enrichment. "Hooked on Phonics" was a newer educational program that was advertised everywhere. Our daycare had used that in conjunction with other tools to teach kids how to read. As corny as the commercial was, it was pretty catchy and memorable; "Hooked on Phonics worked for me!" After participating in just a few classes, the teachers apparently saw a spark in me. I was catching on just as fast as the older kids. They told my parents that I was gifted and although only four years old, was ready to start the first grade. My parents had to really think about this decision. As most parents are, my parents were pretty protective and although they felt I was gifted as well, they wanted to be sure to make the right decision.

Our public school system at that time required an IQ test to consider skipping a grade. Even though kindergarten doesn't seem like much of grade, they considered it one and we had to follow the proper protocol. In general, it was relatively uncommon in our school district to skip a grade and as rare as it was, they didn't have a solid structure for doing so. Each case was considered individually by the school board. So in order for me to start first grade at age five, my parents proceeded with getting an IQ test for me which was conducted by a psychologist who would also evaluate my maturity, as this was a requirement as well.

The car ride seemed like forever. My mom and I were headed to Birmingham, Michigan. It was a suburb of Detroit that wasn't well integrated in the early 90s, or even now for that matter. We rode down Woodward Avenue, a long street that took us from the city to the suburbs.

My mom pulled her blue Ford Tempo into the parking lot of a medium-sized office building. There were several cars in the parking lot. We walked into the lobby and pressed the up button by the elevator bank. Once we got into the office, it was so quiet, you could hear a pin drop. My mom didn't have to warn me to be quiet, as I was quiet-natured by default when I was nervous or in unfamiliar territory. I had no clue what this appointment was going to be like. I knew it was a different type of doctor's appointment—one that did not involve me to take off my clothes and receive shots. I wondered if I would still get a lollipop though.

We sat for about 15 minutes after my mom had checked us in at the front desk. I was fingering through one of the *Highlights* magazines. This was my favorite pastime at the doctor's office. They had the best hidden pictures and I always raced myself to see if I could complete the puzzle before they called my name. *Rooster... rooster. My last picture to find was a rooster and I could not find it! There it is!*

"Tamika Cross," a middle-aged blonde woman was standing in the doorway to the back office. I jumped up and looked at my mom then back at the woman. "You must be Tamika? And this must be your mother?"

My mom responded, "Yes. Can I come back with her?"

"Certainly. We always bring the parents back initially, but once we start testing, we will have to ask you to step out briefly. Is that ok with you, Tamika?" the woman asked. I looked at my mom for approval. I still hadn't opened my mouth once.

"Don't act shy now, Tamika," my mom and the woman chuckled synchronously.

"Yes ma'am. That's fine with me!" I responded. I was excited and scared at the same time. Excited because I loved new challenges and my mom had explained that I may be doing a lot of puzzles and problem solving today. I was also nervous. My parents had told me that this appointment would determine if I could start school or not. Melvin never had to take this test, so I didn't fully understand why I needed to. Having a big brother who was only a couple years older than me made me frequently compare myself to him. If we had dessert, I wanted to know why his piece was bigger. When going to bed, I wanted to know why his bedtime was later. I think it's pretty normal for most siblings to compare themselves to each other. I wasn't upset about having to do this test, I just didn't understand why I had to jump through an extra hoop if no one else had to. I was too young at the time to understand that it was solely because of my age.

We all sat at a round table together that was the perfect height for me. Quite frankly, it seemed pretty short for adults to be sitting at, but I liked that. Finally, something made just for us kids!

"So I understand you were referred here from Southfield Public School Board? You are interested in Tamika starting school a year early, correct?" the psychologist asked my mother.

"Yes. Tamika is performing at a level above her peers and her father and I think that kindergarten would be boring for her. She already knows everything in the kindergarten curriculum. She's very involved in the enrichment classes at her daycare and all of the staff said it would be a complete waste of her time. Her father and I agree," my mom replied.

"Understood. Well, the school board has required an IQ test and psychological evaluation, as you know. The test will not be longer than 45 minutes to an hour. It will be one on one with Tamika and me. I will ask her a series of questions, have her do some activities with matching, shapes, and problem solving. It's pretty straight forward. We do ask that parents step out because we have noticed that children perform better when their parents aren't in the room distracting them. Also, if she is heading to first grade, she will be in school all day without you, so this is a good practice," the doctor explained to my mom.

"Ok. I'll be in the waiting room Tamika," my mom said softly as she grabbed her purse and started for the door slowly. She looked like she didn't want to leave.

We sat in the room for about 45 minutes and the interview went just like the doctor had explained. It seemed pretty simple and it honestly didn't feel like too much of a test. I enjoyed it. Before leaving the office, we stopped at the check out desk and my mom paid for the visit. Apparently, the testing and evaluation was not covered by insurance as it was not medically necessary. My parents had to pay out of pocket. I asked my parents when I got older what made them so pressed to pay out of pocket when they likely weren't rolling in money bags exactly at that time. They both said they felt it was important for me to be challenged and I was bored in preschool and they didn't believe in wasting time. My dad was one of the youngest in his class and my mom who completed high school and college within just three years each, I knew they meant it when they said they weren't interested in wasting time if I was ready. Since the school board made us jump through these couple extra hoops, my parents followed through with it because they felt it was important.

About a week later, my mom received a letter in the mail from the psychologist's office. It included my IQ score and a letter of support for me to skip kindergarten. The next day, my mom went to the Southfield school board while I was at daycare and submitted the results and letter. A few days later, we received a phone call from the school board stating that skipping grades was an unusual circumstance that was not usually supported. However, since we actually went through the processes they listed and my IQ and maturity level supported starting first grade at five, they would allow me start at the school we were zoned to, my brother's school, McIntyre Elementary School. They also explained that this was a trial basis only to see how it went and that we would evaluate after a few months. My mom expressed her understanding and hung up with the lady on the phone. She was excited.

"Well, baby, it looks like you're starting school this fall!" she exclaimed. That moment was special. My parents were always proud of Melvin and me, but in that moment, it felt like I had done something really great. We had a special dinner to celebrate, and my mom was on the phone all night calling family to let them know the great news. I recall asking my parents for my IQ score and they refused to tell me or show me the letter for several years. My parents have always been big on humility and I guess they didn't want me "feeling myself" too much. They told me I scored exceptionally well and that was all I needed to know. I remember asking a million times as a kid what my score was and they refused to tell me. I especially wanted to know when my cousin PJ took an IQ test as well a few years after me. In true kid competitive manner, I wanted to compare scores. PJ was so smart—much smarter than me! He was like a genius in my eyes, so I wanted to see how my score matched up to his. My parents already knew that this is something I would do which even further solidified their decision to not tell me. I was annoyed about it for years, but now as an adult, I completely understand why.

The so called "trial" apparently went well as they never pulled me from the class, never mentioned it again, and I completed first grade and entered in the second grade at age 6, the following year, and so on.

I absolutely loved school. I had an affinity for learning and everyday was exposed to new things. I did frequently find myself bored with the curriculum, though. I finished my work much quicker than other students, then decided to try to teach others while the teacher was talking. I often found myself in trouble for this self-appointed task I had taken on. At parent-teacher conferences, my teachers always had great reports about me as a student and how

I loved to learn. The only complaint to my parents would be "Sometimes, Tamika needs to be reminded that she is not the teacher." My parents would reprimand me about completing my work and being quiet rather than trying to talk over the teachers. It was then that I realized that it was not only learning that I enjoyed, but I even enjoyed teaching others what I had just learned!

When I was in the second grade, my teacher, Ms. Lyons, truly made me love school even more. She was young in her teaching career and fresh out of college. She made learning fun and served as an excellent role model to us. She always believed in me and my success and kept pushing me to the next level when she saw me getting "bored" by the standard curriculum. There was a program in our school district for grades three to five called "Talented and Gifted" program (TAG). She recommended during one of the parent-teacher conferences that I took the test for admission and she would write a letter of recommendation. The only caveat was that at that time, it was available at only one elementary school in the district and that was not my home school. If granted admission, I would have to change to a completely different elementary school. I did not want to leave my friends. I had already been the "new girl" coming in at first grade and everyone else had known each other from kindergarten. Now I was two years in at the same school and I would have to go be the new girl again. My mom explained that since TAG was only at one elementary school, that there would be students in my class from every different elementary school in the district. She reassured me that I would not be the only new girl again and that this would be a more challenging curriculum than what the normal classes had been offering me. I agreed to take the test and was granted admission into the program.

In third grade, I started the TAG program at Stevenson Elementary School. Although I missed my home school, I still saw my friends at after school events and on the school bus. I would take the bus to McIntyre with them, then me and a few others would take a second bus from that school to Stevenson and in the reverse order to go home each day. Navigating the whole taking two buses at seven years old was confusing at first but once I got the hang of it and I did not mind it at all.

I enjoyed TAG. We were always being challenged and functioning one to two grade levels above our grade. We were exposed to different methods of learning and I never once was "bored". The way the TAG program was structured was there was one third grade class, one fourth grade class and one fifth grade class for the entire school district. So you stayed with the same classmates essentially for third through fifth grade (give or take one or two transfers). It was great for establishing friendships with other students because you all would have been together for 3 years straight after completing the TAG program. I still, to this day, keep up with most of my classmates from TAG directly, through mutual friends, or social media.

At the end of third grade, an executive decision from administrators had been made to move the TAG program from Stevenson to Schoenhals Elementary. *A new school AGAIN?* When we moved into a new school, it was not exactly the warmest welcome. Other students continuously picked on us for being "TAG kids", nerds, or the coined nickname of "TAG FAGS". While it did not really bother me surprisingly enough at that age, it sure did get annoying. It made it difficult to make friends outside of your class. Other students did not want to be friends with the "TAG FAGS". They did not want to play with us at recess or sit with us at lunch. Of course, every student was not that way, but many were. We were assumed to be "know-it-alls" and "arrogant" because we had been accepted into the TAG program. I wasn't any of those things. Honestly, I just wanted to hang out, and play the same games they all enjoyed. You almost always expect girls to be catty and divided over silly things, but the guys were that way too. They would play football and basketball with other classes, but they never wanted our TAG boys to be on their team. It was always the TAG boys vs non-TAG boys, etc. I lived near a lot of kids that were zoned to Schoenhals so I made friends at the school from hanging out at the park or riding my bike after school.

Our house was situated on the border of two cities; Lathrup Village and Southfield. When I was attending McIntyre and Stevenson for grades one through three, I was able to catch the bus on the Lathrup Village side. When the TAG program moved to Schoenhals, I could easily walk a block in the opposite direction into Southfield and take the Schoenhals bus. This ended up being easier so I could condense my bus ride down to one bus rather than two. It meant that I was not going to be seeing my friends before and after school anymore, but I would be able to get to school with everyone else, so it was a no brainer for my parents.

At my new bus stop, there was four of us. There was a kindergarten boy named Michael who used to wait for the bus with his grandma and her dog. She was so sweet and always looked over us all to make sure we were safe, or held the bus when one of us was running late. There were two other boys, Theo and Larry who lived nearby and caught the bus at the same stop. Being the only girl at the bus stop did not bother me much, but I guess it made for an easy target to tease.

My brother rode the other bus going to Birney Middle School and this was my first time riding the bus without him. Having an older brother whom I admired, I enjoyed many of the things that he enjoyed—from playing sports, video games, or watching sports. Being that he was only two years older than me, I frequently wore his "hand-me-down" clothes. Back in the 90s, denim baggy jeans and plaid shirts were in style. I didn't mind taking his clothes that didn't fit anymore. I would take his jeans and cut them into shorts, or tie his baggy shirts around my waist, etc. I wore "girly" clothes too, but I had a pretty broad style. One day I would wear a dress, another day an Isiah Thomas jersey with gym shoes, denim overalls, and boots the next day. I liked the versatility in my style.

Sometimes, I got sick of the hand-me-downs from my big brother. He would get more new clothes and I would get his gently used clothes. I would still get new clothes too, but not as much as he did. He was a "rapidly growing boy" who was quickly growing out of the clothes and shoes my parents would buy each year. For the most part, wearing Melvin's clothes wasn't a bad thing. I created my own style with them and I was comfortable with that.

One day at the bus stop, I had on some denim shorts I had cut from his jeans, a University of Michigan tee shirt and my Fila gym shoes. I was relatively shy at the bus stop. I was at a new school, at a new bus stop, and was with all boys. I quietly waited for the bus. Theo and Larry were behind me snickering. I had no idea about what nor did I turn around to investigate.

"Why do you always look like a boy?" Theo asked me. Larry burst into laughter.

"Yeah, you always are wearing your brother's baggy clothes. Can y'all not afford any more clothes and you have to share?" Larry inquired.

I remained silent.

"Seriously, when you wear your hair like that too, sometimes I think you're a boy. And those big glasses make you look so ugly!" Theo added.

The bus pulled up, I got on the bus and sat with a friend. I ignored them the remainder of the bus ride. After school,

I rode the bus home and when it pulled up at my stop, I jumped off the steps and started on my way home. Larry and Theo followed me for a few houses, taunting remarks that were a continuation from that morning. I went home and acted unbothered and did not share the story with my family. This continued on for several weeks and one day I cracked.

My brother was in middle school now and he got home from school earlier than I did. I walked into the house and put my bags down and headed to my room. My normal routine was to use the bathroom, then ask my brother for a snack and we would watch after school shows and do our homework until our parents came home from work. I didn't want a snack that day. My brother came in my bedroom asking me what I wanted for a snack only to find me face down on my bed crying.

"What's wrong, TT? Is everything ok?" he asked, concerned.

"I hate my new school! They keep making fun of me at the bus stop!" I reported back in between tears.

"Who is making fun of you? Why haven't you told me?" Melvin jumped into protective big brother mode. "Where are they at? I'll handle them!"

"The boys at the bus stop have been making fun of me every day! They say I am ugly and look like a boy. They keep calling me poor saying I have to share clothes with my big brother!" I sniffled. After Melvin calmed me down like only he could do, we developed a plan that he would meet me at the bus stop the next day and have a "talk" with them. I couldn't wait.

The very next day, as soon as the bus pulled up to let us off after school, I saw my big brother waiting there. I was smiling from ear to ear. They'll be sure to leave me alone now. I hop off the bus. Larry wasn't on the bus that day, maybe he had been picked up from school. Theo was there by himself. My brother approached him within seconds of him getting off the bus.

"Hey are you Theo?" Melvin asked, already knowing who he was based on the description I had given him as the "tall one."

"Yea, why what's up man?" Theo asked with his voice quivering. Theo was tall, but my brother was much taller and bigger in general.

"You need to leave my little sister alone. She told me y'all have been picking on her since she's been coming over here and it needs to stop!" He said firmly. Theo started bawling pretty hysterically. Wow. That was not at all what I expected. My brother had been firm and direct but had not laid a finger on him. For some reason I felt really bad at that moment. I felt like a bully. I told Melvin that it was enough and we should go home.

Theo stayed there surprisingly. He didn't run, or try to fight my brother. He just cried like a baby. I felt horrible. This boy had been bullying me since I came to the school and acted big and bad with his friends around and when my brother said a few words to him he is literally crying like a baby. I knew at that moment how weak he truly was, as most bullies are on the inside. I didn't want us to stoop to his level. I yanked on Melvin's arm begging him to leave and then my tears started coming down my face. Melvin stopped and looked at me with a look of disgust.

"T, what are you crying for?" He asked.

"I just wanted you to scare him a little bit but I didn't want to make anyone cry!" At that point, I was bawling like Theo. My brother shook me off his arm and stomped home. I ran behind him asking him why was he mad at me. He ignored me and kept walking. Mom was at home when we got back to the house. She knew that he was helping me "sort some things out" at the bus stop. She opened the door.

"Melvin why do you look mad and Tamika, why on earth are you crying?" My mom was perplexed.

"Mannnnnn, Tamika likes that kid! What a complete waste of my time! Tamika don't ask me for anything else! How are you going to start crying with the guy? I'm on your side! You like that dude!" he shouted.

"I don't like him, but I don't like making people cry! I didn't know he was going to cry! I felt bad!" I defended myself. My mom was laughing. This incident is a forever laughing point in our family and they make fun of me for it. To this day, they think I had a secret crush on Theo and there's nothing I can say to make them two feel otherwise.

I couldn't stand him. He bullied me and made me feel ashamed of the clothes I wore and how I looked. It wasn't the type of teasing like a boy does when he likes a girl. It was mean, hurtful things that I eventually learned to ignore. I truly just didn't want to make this boy cry. I knew he had other insecurities and I genuinely felt bad for him. He called me poor, ugly, a tomboy—you name it. He stopped after the day he met Melvin. His buddy Larry would consider himself "roasting" me, but Theo rarely joined in anymore. He knew that if he crossed me, I could easily "out" him as the crying little punk he was on the inside.

Although I was only nine years old, I knew that this was a sign of a deeper-rooted issue within himself. Later on in the school year, I realized that his mom was having financial hardships, and it was publicly known when they were evicted from the house they were living in. All off their belongings from his sports trophies, to their clothes to their beds were thrown out on their front lawn for the neighborhood to see. Fragile items were broken into pieces. We all knew that it meant that someone had been evicted. Although he made fun of my family and called us poor, and made it a point to tease me every single day about it, in actuality, they weren't exactly well off either.

Neighborhood kids teased him and talked about him for months. I genuinely felt bad for him and his family. Kids can be so cruel and although he made my transition to a new school horrible, not once did I think I would feel comforted by seeing his family publicly go through that. The foundation behind bullying is almost always built on insecurities. I realized that a young age and it stuck with me for years to come when trying to navigate past negative words and energy.

Once the bullying from the bus stop was behind me, the remainder of fourth and fifth grade got better. I had made a lot of friends at the new school even outside the TAG program. I was beginning to like the school and not feel so out of place. The girls in the other classes weren't as bad as they had initially seemed when they were hesitant to befriend us.

After lunch, many of us girls would go to the bathroom before heading back to class. There was a bathroom at the end of our hallway and girls from the three fifth grade classes used the same one. My friend Arica and I stopped in the bathroom after lunch one day only to find the usual after lunch bathroom clique in there. They were making spit balls and putting them on the ceiling. They made them with water and toilet paper and shot them up to the ceiling where they would stick. I looked up at the ceiling to find hundreds of old spit balls that were hardened on the ceiling. The girls were adding to the collection. It seemed dumb and pointless to me and I didn't understand what was so exciting about this activity. Arica and I headed to the mirror and sink at the back of the bathroom to apply our lip gloss. She and I used the same 99-cent lip gloss from the beauty supply store. My favorite "flavor" was cherry, and so was hers. We used to see who could apply the most lip gloss for the shiniest lips. While this contest seems silly now, it was way more fun than throwing spit balls on the ceiling and destroying school property. One of the girls grabbed our attention.

"Do you guys know how to throw a spit ball?" she asked.

"Um, not really. We aren't interested in learning either," I replied and stared blankly.

"Come on... y'all TAG FAGs are such goodie two shoes. You're scared to get in trouble? It's no big deal," the ring leader pressed us.

"We aren't scared to get in trouble. We just don't want to do it!" Arica stammered.

"Just try one. It's really easy." she said.

We ended up succumbing to the peer pressure and attempted to land a spit ball on the ceiling. Neither of them stuck to the ceiling, and came tumbling down on the floor. We grabbed our failed spit ball off the floor and tossed in the trash. The other girls continued with the spit balls on the ceiling. Another girl walked in the bathroom. She looked concerned with what they were doing but didn't open up her mouth. Arica and I left the bathroom.

Later that day, we got called to the principal's office. The girl who walked in at the end had reported all of us for destroying school property. They questioned the other girls and they reassured them that it was only me and my friend throwing spit balls and that we were trying to vandalize the school because we were in TAG and not feeling welcomed. We explained that we had thrown spit balls once and they fell on the ground and we threw it in the trash. They did not believe us. Arica and I had to stay after school and using a broom and a ladder, remove every single spit ball, new, old, etc.

The other girls ratted us out and flipped the entire story. We were in the wrong place at the wrong time and the entire incident was blamed on us. This was confirmation that the company you keep makes all the difference. Regardless if any of the remaining spit balls were mine, I was caught in the act and would be punished accordingly. I was so mad at myself for allowing them to pressure us into something we had no desire of doing anyways. This was another formative transition that taught me to stand my ground and never let someone peer pressure me into making a decision or doing something that is not aligned with my morals and core values.

After the TAG program was completed and when we graduated fifth grade, we went to the same middle school as everyone else. There were three options in our school system. They had honors math classes for us to continue down that accelerated path, but every other subject there were not any honors classes. That seemed to be lacking. If in fifth grade, we were reading and writing at the sixth and seventh grade level—what did they expect us to do in the sixth grade? They had not thought that all the way through I suppose...

A few of the TAG students went to private schools to be able to continue at the accelerated level. My parents were not sending me to a private school, nor did I want to attend one. I just was happy to be normal again. At least I wouldn't be ostracized anymore because, although there were a couple honors/AP classes, there was not a TAG program that divided students at the middle and high school levels.

Being in TAG definitely started me on my accelerated trajectory that continued through high school honors/AP classes, graduating in the top 10% of my high school, matriculating into a top tier university on full scholarship and landing myself a spot in medical school all by the age of 20. There may have been a few bumps on the road along the way, a few years of jokes and taunting, but I don't regret being a TAG kid at all. I do believe that attending three different elementary schools taught me social skills and how to adapt quickly to new settings; a characteristic that has worked in my favor into my adulthood.

Affirmation to recite: *What may seem as a handicap now, can end up being a blessing later. I am comfortable being me.*

Question: *Can you recall a time that you were teased for the very thing that ended up being a blessing later on in your life?*

CHAPTER 3

A Dream Deferred

"What happens to a dream deferred? Does it dry up like a raisin in the sun? Or does it explode?"

—Langston Hughes

"Tamika, we received a letter in the mail on your behalf. Do you know what this is about?" my dad asked, fingering through the mail he grabbed from the mailbox on his way in from work.

"No Daddy, why would I?" I questioned.

"You know we don't like surprises. You didn't get in trouble at school lately did you?" his eyebrow raised.

"No dad! Why do y'all always ask that? I already know the consequences I'm up against! I haven't gotten in trouble in a while!" I whined. For the past couple years, end of middle school and start of high school, I had a few behavioral struggles in school. I received a few detentions and suspensions for various things. The underlying issue was usually my smart mouth. Today we call them clapbacks, but boy did I have a natural supply ready to fire anytime I was challenged.

One thing I'm not and have never been is a liar. Anytime I was called out for something I didn't do or wasn't responsible for, rather than being quiet, I made it a point to say what I felt. Being expressive as a kid was a blessing and a curse. Pent up emotions and feelings are never encouraged but speaking out every time wasn't either. As my dad would frequently remind me, "Tamika, you don't have to always have the last word." I was an academically phenomenal student in middle school with a hefty file of behavioral modifications. When I started high school, my parents were really regretting me staying in our public school system. They didn't feel it was challenging me enough and they felt I needed more structure. My parents wanted me in private school since I started but couldn't afford it back then. Now after building a strong academic record, they were able to look into possibilities of scholarships to some of the top private schools in the state. I was uninterested. I was sick of being ostracized (with the other smart kids) all the time. I didn't want to be in a special program and special school. I just wanted to have fun and do crazy stuff with my friends. My parents pulled my brother Melvin from the public school system after middle school. They felt like he needed more structure and focus as well. They enrolled him at the University of Detroit Jesuit High School which was an all-boys Catholic school. He wasn't thrilled at first, but when it was time for me to go to high school, he had already navigated his first two years.

"TT, it ain't that bad, honestly. It sucks at first but you get used to it. You can still see your friends after school!" he encouraged. My parents wanted me to attend the all-girls sister school of the school that he attended. They made me do a tour and spend a day there to check the school out. I was completely tuned out. At 13 years old, I was all into boys—why would I want to go to an all-girls school. Melvin's girlfriend at the time went there and she used to share way too many stories of girls hitting on girls in the bathroom. I don't know if they were true or not, but I was not feeling it at all. I begged my parents to let me stay in the public school system. They agreed, as long as I cleaned up my behavior.

My mom was working for Detroit Public Schools at the time and she was a fan of Cass Technological High School or Renaissance High School for me. She felt although DPS got a bad reputation with the school system at times, she knew firsthand that these schools were good and arguably better than the school I wanted to attend with my friends. There was a year-long debate and back and forth in my family. The final verdict was that my parents would let me go to Southfield Lathrup High School with my friends, but the first time I got in trouble, they were pulling me from the school and sending me to an all-girls private school. That was enough for me to bite my tongue. So my dad asking if this was a disciplinary letter from the school was somewhat warranted. I knew I wasn't in trouble though.

"Open the letter! I promise I haven't gotten in trouble!" I exclaimed.

"It isn't a bill from something else you ordered either, is it?" my mom shot me a quick look.

"Ha ha ha! Very funny! I don't even remember that! This family will never let me forget that incident, huh?" I questioned. When I was 4 years old, and just learning how to read, there was a Disney commercial advertising the channel. For all of my younger readers, the Disney channel did not come with regular cable back in the day. It was a premium channel that had to be paid for separately like HBO or Showtime. There was a commercial showing all the best cartoons that would be on the Disney channel and I wanted it! At the end of the commercial there was a number to call if interested in ordering the channel. I picked up the phone while my parents were in the other room and I called and ordered the Disney channel. Why they took an order from a four year old, I have no clue. But they added the channel to our cable package. My brother and I would watch all the shows on the Disney channel and enjoyed it immensely. My parents didn't find out about it until it showed up on the next bill. I got in trouble, but they didn't cancel the channel. They were more so amazed at how I was able to do that at 4 years old. This is one of the biggest running jokes in my family. They knew I was going to be a handful when I was ordering things via telephone at four!

My parents finally opened the letter. It was a letter informing me that I had been nominated for the National Youth Leadership Forum on Medicine (NYLF). Wow, I didn't know what the program was but being nominated for something seemed like quite the honor. It was a ten-day program that exposed rising eleventh grade students to a career in medicine. I had dreamed of becoming a doctor since I was in elementary school so I was elated.

Who nominated me for this? When does it start? Where was this program at? Apparently, the program was at multiple locations, none of which were in Michigan. So if I wanted to attend the program, I would have to travel out of state for the ten-day duration. I had never been out of state before without my parents. My parents and I looked at the brochure to see what locations I could choose from. As I scanned the list, my eyes shot directly to Emory University in Atlanta, Georgia. I didn't know much about Emory but the little I had known about the school made me interested in attending there for medical school! They were one of the top programs in the country right in the heart of Atlanta.

"Look mom, they have Emory on the list! I want to go to that location!" I shouted, more excitedly than a kid in a candy store.

"Well hold on, we have to look over the brochure more, see the cost, and your father and I have to talk about it," she said.

"Ok! Well let's circle Emory, because that's the one I want to go to, just in case you guys forget!" I responded. Typical Tamika, excited beyond measure and a planner down to every detail. I wanted to make sure they didn't forget which location I was interested in so circling the location would help them when it was time to register me! I was that kid; the busybody kid who wanted to participate in every extracurricular activity there was. At that time, I was already in dance, captain of the varsity tennis team, the student board secretary, recently quit the swim team, in Girl Scouts, National Honor Society, Scholars Plus, and on the Step Team. I know I kept my parents busy and their pockets empty. They rarely told me no when I wanted to do something because they felt it was important to allow me to spread my wings and explore new things. I wanted to be in everything! This NYLF program was for my career and since it was academically based, I knew there was no way they wouldn't let me go.

After a few days of them reviewing the materials and discussing among each other, they sat me down. "Tamika, come in here so we can talk to you." My mom yelled while I was finishing my homework before dinner. My dad usually was at work until pretty late but today he was home a little earlier. I walked into the living room where they both were sitting. Oh wow, I must be in trouble, I thought.

"You're not in trouble, T. Just have a seat." My dad reassured me.

"So we have been looking at this program you want to go to in Atlanta. It looks like a really nice program and it is this summer in July. It's already March and enrollment is taking place in the next month. The cost is way outside of our means right now and we know how much you want to go. Unfortunately, we aren't going to be able to do it this year," he said in an unusually quiet tone.

"But please! I will drop some of my other activities to help with the cost! I really want to go!" I cried.

"Tamika, we just don't have it, baby," My mom said looking like she was on the verge of tears. My parents were the hardest workers I had ever seen and they made every effort to be able to allow Melvin and I to participate in whatever we wanted. I knew if they could have paid for it, they would have. The look in their eyes was one of defeat. They looked as if they had let me down in telling me no. I felt horrible. *How selfish can I be? They said they didn't have it and there I was trying to convince them.* Although I was entering the eleventh grade, and most of my friends were 16, I had just turned 15. I was too young for a driver's license and too young to work unless I wanted to bag groceries at Kroger. I needed a job that made more money than that. I braided hair on the side but I didn't make enough to pay for a $2000 program. I had to accept that I was not going to be able to go and make a huge effort to not make my parents feel like crap about it either.

"Yeah, I understand. I was scared to leave the state by myself anyways," I lied. My best friend, Deonna had been nominated for the same program and her parents were paying for her to go. We would have been able to room together. She spent her summers in Alabama so her parents would be driving her to Atlanta rather than flying from Detroit, but once we were there we would have been inseparable. We had already planned out what stuff we would be taking and we couldn't wait. They told us we would have been staying in college dorms at Emory so we were excited to have a college experience at such a young age.

How was I going to tell her that I wasn't going anymore? I guess I never was told that I was going, but in my head I just knew that I was and in typical narcissistic teenager fashion, I had spilled the beans that I was going.

Money didn't ever seem to be as tight in her family, so I knew she was going to be able to go. Honestly, I did have a few flashes of jealousy over the years when I would see her decked out in expensive designer clothes, purses, and shoes. It was normal at that age, but I felt bad for feeling that way. I had the best parents a kid could ask for so when I had those moments I used to quickly wash them out of my mind.

A few weeks went by and I had already broken the news to Deonna. She didn't even want to go anymore if I wasn't going to be there with her. But as an aspiring doctor as well, her parents encouraged her participation regardless if I would be there or not. My mom called me into her room one day to inform me that I would be able to go to Atlanta that summer.

"Your uncle Steve and grandpa have split the bill and sponsored your entire trip for the ten days. You better call them both up now and thank them for this!" my mom said. My mom never asked either of them to pay for the program, and knowing her pride, she never would have. She had shared with her mom, my grandmother, that I had been accepted into this program and how much I wanted to do it. She also shared with my grandmother that they couldn't afford it and felt horrible about letting me down.

Apparently, my grandmother spoke to my uncle and grandpa about it and within seconds they both had agreed to pay for the trip. Both of them being college professors truly valued my affinity for school and learning and they wanted me to be able to attend this program as they felt it would positively influence and support my decision to one day become a doctor. I thanked them both profusely with a phone call and a typed up letter I wrote upon completion of the program. My letter included all the things we did and why I was appreciative of the program and them sending me there.

Prior to attending the program, I had no idea how engulfed in medicine I truly would be during those ten days. My love for medicine and dream of becoming a doctor stemmed from my grandmother. She was a registered nurse and she shared so many amazing stories from nursing school to working as a nurse in the hospital for years later. She made the medical field sound fun yet so rewarding. From hearing her stories growing up to also seeing the perspective as my grandmother being the patient, it was very clear to me how I wanted to leave my mark in this world. I spent so much time with my grandmother growing up; we were essentially inseparable. She understood me in a way that I felt no one else did. Even when I went off to college, sometimes I would be going through a tough time, call her up at 3 AM, because I knew she was up, and just hold the phone. She knew I was crying, stressed, frustrated and that her presence even through the phone was consoling enough for me to make it through the night.

My grandmother was a second mother to me and I never imagined life without her, as I'm sure most children don't at that age. We often feel like our loved ones are going to be around forever and can take our precious time with them for granted. My grandmother and I did everything together; from watching TV, going through old pictures and trinkets, writing poems, playing board games or cards, to attending the majority of her doctor visits with her. Going to the doctor may not sound like an exciting pastime for a kid, but I enjoyed it a great deal. All her doctors came to know me very well. I knew which ones she loved and which ones she dreaded seeing.

My grandmother was a brittle diabetic. As a result of her diabetes, she had kidney, heart, circulation, and nerve issues all that required a different specialist. I watched my grandmother check her blood sugar regularly, administer insulin to herself, and adjust her diet accordingly. I knew that going over her house would involve me eating sugar free candy and sugar free ice cream. I'm sure she wouldn't have minded buying my brother and I whatever we wanted, but it didn't taste that different so we didn't mind it. We watched the multiple hospitalizations over the years and knew the symptoms of hypoglycemia or low blood sugar very well. By the age of 12, I already knew from experience, the signs and symptoms of diabetic ketoacidosis like the back of my hand. Every time I watched my grandmother being carried away on a stretcher by an EMS crew, I knew that she would be in the hospital for a little while.

While many kids develop a fear of the hospital because of the brain associations made—death and illness among others—I wasn't afraid of the hospital. While I hated seeing any close family members hospitalized, it didn't do the same thing to me that it did to most people. I wanted to see everything. What medicine are they hanging, how are they drawing blood, did the doctors conversation make sense, did they stand over my grandmother when they talked, or did they sit down in a chair to be at the same level. Some doctors seemed to be in a rush to either head home or to the next patient, while others sat down, crossed their legs, and answered my grandmother's questions along with my mothers.

Even at a young age, these are things I was paying attention to. I soon learned that the ones who knew my name stayed awhile and talked with my grandmother and asked about her other family members were always her favorite. The doctors she didn't care for too much were always so condescending, rude, and the entire encounter felt rushed. I took mental notes, even if I didn't realize at that age that it would play a major role in the bedside manner I would exude as a practicing physician.

July 6, 2003, my parents drove me to the Detroit airport. The day had finally come for me to head to Atlanta for the NYLF program at Emory. I was filled with excitement and a little bit of fear. I had never been out of state without my parents and I surely had never flown on an airplane by myself. With my mom previously working for the airlines, we had flown a lot as kids and I knew the process in and out but it would be different to navigate it alone. I was 15 years old and felt like I was grown so I would never let anyone see the fear that I truly had. My best friend Deonna was attending the program with me but since she was spending the summer in Alabama with her family, they were driving her to Atlanta as it was a relatively short car ride away. I knew that if I had acted scared, this may impede other summer programs and trips I may want to go on, so I knew I had to keep my poker face on around my parents.

The plane ride wasn't too bad and Deonna and her parents met me at the airport and took us to the meeting location at Emory. We were both excited to be in Atlanta and spending the next ten days with other students that shared the same affinity for medicine as us. Once we arrived and sat through a long orientation, we were able to unpack in our dorm room. This excited us way too much.

Looking back on college, I was never that excited about tiny, dirty dorm rooms with shared bathrooms and mediocre food. But at age 15, it all seemed exhilarating to be on a real college campus and staying in a dorm room like we went to college. Deonna and I had planned to try to blend in with the college students and venture off to see what college life really entailed. That was an unrealistic plan, as the ten-day agenda was packed with activities with 300 other students. We had to wear an ID badge everywhere we went to identify us as high school students in the NYLF program. This was majorly throwing off our plan of "blending in" with the Emory college students. Nonetheless, we partnered off in groups for various activities throughout the program. Deonna and I unfortunately were not paired off in the same group. It forced us to socialize with other people and make new friends.

Each group did different things, but many of the activities were overlapping to ensure a similar experience for all students. When we were all together, they introduced the group of residents who would be working with us and giving us tours of the school and Grady Memorial Hospital. Grady is one of the most well-known hospitals in Atlanta known for their trauma. It was said multiple times during this program that anyone who had been shot or stabbed, Grady was where you wanted to go. They dealt with it so much that many of the staff there could tend to these major issues with their eyes closed.

When they introduced all the residents, I remember eyeballing a Black female resident who seemed to be well accomplished. There she stood in front of all of us telling us about her path in becoming a doctor and she looked just like me! I wanted to be like her already and I barely knew much more than her name and a snippet of her resume. When we paired off into groups, I was ecstatic to be assigned to her group! She seemed like a great resident to follow around and she wasn't uptight and stuck up. Not that the other residents were, but I always had this mental image based on others saying how doctors acted, and she was nothing like that. She was down to earth, cool, laid back, approachable, and highly intelligent. I really wanted to be just like her one day!

Our first activity involved us learning how to suture on a banana. *Why are we using fruit to practice suturing? I thought we would be sewing up real people! Did I fly all the way to Atlanta to practice "doctoring" on a piece of fruit that sat on my kitchen counter back home?* Although these thoughts went through my head, I wouldn't dare say them out loud—well, at that age anyways. She began to explain that the skin on a banana is very similar to human skin so if we could sew up a banana well without unequal tension, then we would have no problem on human skin. Ok, fair enough, if this would help me and my suture skills, then great.

I didn't really know how much pediatricians actually suture, and that's what I had wanted to do since I was a kid, but it was worth the experience. We did use real sutures and needles and needle drivers—the instrument used to hold the needle while a surgeon is suturing a patient. I've always had great dexterity and this activity came pretty easy to me. My first couple of passes, I was pulling too tight to make it perfect. I was quickly reminded by the resident that suturing isn't quite like sewing up a shirt, and that if I pulled too tight, I could either break the suture and have to start all over, or cause more pain to patient or even worse, cut off the blood supply to the surrounding tissue impeding healing and potentially causing a worse issue than a mere laceration. I took her advice and did not pull as hard on my next pass. She explained that entering the tissue (banana skin) at a 90-degree angle is the best technique and showed us the simple movement of twisting our wrist to pass the needle smoothly through the skin. After a few passes, I was definitely feeling myself. I could get the hang of this.

When we finished, she complemented my banana that had evenly spaced sutures with equal tension and it was a very pretty appearance. The perfectionist in me couldn't stop smiling from ear to ear. I wanted to sew up a few more bananas and keep practicing at home. It was time for our next activity, and I didn't want to leave this one. This was probably my earliest age of planting a seed that I may actually want to go into a field where I would be operating. I told our resident just that.

"Brianna, thanks for showing us how to suture! That was so fun! I thought I wanted to be a pediatrician but they probably don't get to sew up people a lot, do they? I think I may want to be a surgeon!" I exclaimed.

"Tamika, where are you from?" she said as she looked closer at my name badge that read Detroit, Michigan. "Detroit, huh? Your family sent you all the way down here to participate in this program? That's pretty cool! I'm glad you enjoyed the suturing simulation lab. There are a lot of different doctors that suture outside of being a surgeon. Of course, if you want to be a surgeon, you can do that too. But know that they spend many hours in the operating room, and they get a lot deeper than just sewing up skin. Not everyone can stomach it."

"Thanks! Yeah, they knew I really wanted to participate in this program! What can't they stomach? Seeing people cut open and the blood that comes along with it? Is that what you think I'm afraid of?"

"Well, no I'm not speaking of you specifically, but I'm just saying there's a lot more to being a surgeon than sewing up skin. We will be passing by the operating room later. Maybe we can take a quick peek so I can show you what I mean!" she stated.

"Oh, I would love that!" I exclaimed. *This trip was getting better and better. I didn't know if peeking into the operating room was part of the schedule, but I was so happy that Brianna was making it a part of ours.* All of us were excited for when the time would come. We toured Grady from the ER to the patient rooms, to the resident call rooms. It was a busy hospital and we saw trauma after trauma being rolled into the ER while we were downstairs. That was when I saw what everyone meant when they said this is the place to go for trauma.

What I noticed about this hospital was that most of the patients were Black or Hispanic. Grady is the public hospital in Atlanta and is the 5th largest public hospital in the country. It is known for being one of the busiest Level I trauma centers in the US. The patient population is mainly comprised of low income, indigent patients. As an academic site, it is staffed with doctors and residents from Emory University as well as Morehouse School of Medicine. As we walked around on our tour, I felt like I was watching an episode of ER. The fast-paced environment with doctors and nurses having conversations at the nurses' stations and performing walking rounds as a team.

Walking rounds is something that every academic program does daily, sometimes two or three times a day depending on the specialty. It is similar to morning report, except we walked as a multi-disciplinary team to present each patient and check in on them. The team would consist of nurses, attending physicians, resident physicians, medical students, social workers, dieticians, etc., and discuss each patient one at a time. This is also a time for teaching or what many medical professionals refer to as "pimping". Typically, the attending physician, who is the leader of the team will start with asking a difficult question to the medical student, if he or she does not know the answer, it will go to the intern, or first-year resident, and if they are stumped, an upper level resident would be expected to answer correctly. If no one on the team can answer the question correctly, the chief resident is typically held responsible.

The chief resident is a resident in their final year of training who was elected by peers and faculty to be the leader of the program. Some programs have one chief, some have two or three; it really depends on the size of the program. Depending on your attending, rounds could be fun or very stressful. Every attending has different teaching techniques. You have the belittling, dramatic, nonchalant, laid-back, or hard ass attending.

The belittling attending will humiliate you in front of the team in effort to engrain the experience in your head to make sure you never forget again. While this method works for some learners, it truly makes some learners shut down and hold a grudge. As a person who always had somewhat of an inappropriate sense of humor, these attendings always made rounds interesting and comical. Of course it's not funny when you're in the hot seat, but when Brad is being chewed out for not listening to a patient's lung sounds at 6 AM, it makes for light entertainment at the start of the day.

The dramatic attendings are the ones who make the biggest deal out of the smallest thing. Now I will admit, what we all thought was small as a student and as a resident, may not be what I see as small today as a practicing physician. An example of that is when an attending would go crazy over a male medical student not having on a tie or having on a wrinkled white lab coat. It was stupid to me back then, but I soon realized that presentation is everything and "looking the part" and being professional goes a long way for not only your staff and colleagues, but for your patients. This was drilled in especially when I was in medical school at Meharry. Most of us were minorities and as unfortunate as it may be, they shared the harsh reality that without us looking the part, we would frequently be overlooked and passed over and mistaken as another profession or a patient's family member. Unbeknownst to me at that time, the whitest, crispest white coat with starched creases and a name badge that reads "DOCTOR" may still not be enough depending on the color of your skin or your gender. But I digress...

Minor details are very important in many cases as they impact the care of the patient, and attention to detail is an important characteristic that a good physician should harbor. But the dramatic attendings focus on things like if you printed their patient list in portrait format instead of landscape like they prefer to leave room in the margins for notes. Now I always understood that everyone has a preference and if the attending likes it a certain way, then we should honor that. The dramatic attending yells about this for an hour, wasting everyone's time because Sarah printed the list the wrong way by accident. It could easily be fixed by having her go print a new list and moving on to the next patient. But to spend an hour talking about how Sarah does what Sarah wants to do and how Sarah doesn't follow directions or doesn't care about being a physician, is a little bit... dramatic!

The nonchalant attendings are the one who show up to rounds as a necessity for their job description, but is really ready to move on to something else. They aren't picking on your presentation or "pimping" you about the causes of a deep venous thrombosis either. He or she shows up to rounds, rushes your presentation, usually only wants to hear from the chief and is ready to move on. While some days it's refreshing to have the nonchalant attending because you know rounds will be quick and you won't get cursed out for not reading up on your patients medical conditions by 7 AM after being assigned the patients at 6 AM and having to see them and finish notes within an hour, you didn't learn much on those days. I never enjoyed those rounds. I always wanted to learn something from rounds even if it meant I would be in the hot seat and humiliated for the morning. I felt like these attendings didn't care, and while I don't know that to be fact, I always felt that these attendings didn't belong in academic medicine. They would be better off in private practice where they can see patients and be efficient, rather than taking the time to teach young learners.

The laid-back attending is different from the nonchalant attending. These attendings show that they care and are invested in the resident and student education and learning. They just are much nicer in their approach. These are the attendings who show up with breakfast or coffee because they knew that none of us weren't able to squeeze in breakfast before a long rounding session. They also had an approach to learning that was helpful but a little more sugar coated. With knowing firsthand the stressors in the life of a medical student and resident, they didn't want to make it worse—if anything, they wanted to build you up after you spent the last week being broken down by the job, lack of sleep, patient demands, and academic expectations.

Last but not least is the hard ass attending. They nitpick everything you say, but it's warranted and legit. They are like a walking textbook and know medicine like the back of their hand and hold you to the same high standard no matter if it's your first month being a doctor or you're a graduating resident four years later. They are hard on you, but not in a demeaning way. They push you to be a better physician. I always gravitated to these attendings. They felt like a personal trainer who pisses you off when they tell you ten more seconds on the plank only to realize that in those ten seconds, there are six ones, six twos, six threes... and before you know it you've been holding the plank for an extra 60 seconds! It's annoying as hell but your abs thank you later when you begin seeing results.

That's how I categorize the hard ass attendings. You always have to be on your Ps and Qs, but if you're prepared, well read, and on top of your shit, they will give you a praise or two. An example of this was on my OBGYN rotation at Meharry when my attending had me see a postpartum patient and present her. She had delivered several weeks prior but was still having some vaginal discharge but it wasn't bloody anymore. My inquisitive self asked my attending during rounds why she had whitish yellow discharge coming out now. Instead of her answering my question, she made me stay after class that day to look it up in a textbook and report back to her. My classmates laughed and joked as they walked out while I'm sitting here fingering through a 1000-page textbook trying to find out why this patient had whitish yellow discharge coming from her vagina postpartum.

I ended up giving her a full report about lochia and the different types of lochia and how long the patient experiences lochia rubra, lochia serosa, and lochia alba. Some may think this was super extra and she could have just answered my question, but I honestly appreciated that extraness. There I was asking a question that I could have easily looked up. I never forgot about this story or about the different types of lochia, as I am writing about this story from over ten years ago like it happened yesterday. The teaching method must have worked, because it stuck!

Beyond teaching me about the different types of lochia, it taught me how to be resourceful which is useful as a doctor. In medicine, you don't have to know everything about everything but you have to at least know where to go to find the answer, and discovering that truth has made a huge difference in my career.

We continued on our tour. We visited the morgue and saw amputated limbs and dead fetuses in containers. It was quite graphic to many students who couldn't wait to move on, but I was intrigued. I was really enjoying myself. We made a lot of noise as we moved through the busy hospital, from the talking amongst each other to the clicking of our business casual shoes we had on. Patients in the hallway stopped and stared as we roamed the busy hallways of Grady Memorial. When we got upstairs to where the operating rooms were, Brianna looked at me and signaled for me to come to the front.

I frequently walked toward the back of the group because I enjoyed taking it all in and looking around. Sometimes my amazement had me fall behind the group a bit and I didn't want to hold others up. I never let the group out of sight, but I enjoyed looking around and envisioning myself here in a few years. *I could do this. I would make a great doctor. I could get the hang of this and walk the halls with the same level of confidence as these other doctors. I wanted to be like Brianna.* She seemed to know everyone from the nursing staff, to doctors in other specialties, she was like a hospital celebrity. I walked up to the front as Brianna directed.

"Tamika, this is where they have all the operating rooms. My friend is a surgery resident as well and he said he is about to scrub in on a surgery called an incision and drainage. You cannot really see from out here, unfortunately. Without proper attire, you cannot even go back there to watch closer either," she said.

"Well how can I know if I want to be a surgeon without going into the operating room?" I asked, "I want to watch the surgery, is that allowed?"

"Without scrubs, a surgical mask, and hat, you cannot go back there, Tamika. Maybe next time," she said softly. *Next time? When would I ever get an experience like this? I almost didn't make it down here for this program and I wanted to maximize my experience.* This was characteristic of me then and still is now. I liked to push the limits. How far can I go? Closed mouths don't get fed. It won't hurt to ask, so I wanted to see how to get myself in that operating room.

"Well I saw that resident grab scrubs from over there, can someone maybe get me a pair? And the hat and masks are over there by the sink. Please, can I go in the surgery?" I already had planned out the whole thing within seconds. My mind was made up and I didn't care how much the other students saw me grabbling. Well, it worked. They found me scrubs, a bouffant for my hair, a surgical mask, and asked the group if anyone else wanted to come in and watch the surgery. Surprisingly only one other student wanted to go in the actual OR. They were missing out!

I went to the bathroom and put on the scrubs. I always took forever getting dressed in the morning, my parents can attest to that. I put on those scrubs in less than a minute and darted out of the bathroom to find Brianna. The group was waiting just outside the doors for her. The surgery was starting and she urged me and the other student to go inside the operating room now. The O.R. nurse instructed for us to stand back away from the sterile field. It was taped off and all blue and we couldn't touch anything near that because we were not sterile.

The process of becoming sterile includes first wearing hospital assigned and laundered scrubs, washing your hands with special soap for 3 minutes, drying off with sterile towels in a technique that goes from your hand to your elbow being sure to use different sides of the towel for each hand, then with the assistance of a surgical tech who was already gowned and sterile, putting on a gown and gloves. The technique seemed seamless but there were a lot of steps and one wrong step can make you become unsterile and have to go back outside and start the entire process over again. We had to learn this technique when we were third year medical students and if we didn't have it downpacked, we would get yelled at and more than likely not be able to scrub in for the surgery. It was a big deal to properly know the technique of washing and dressing in a sterile fashion, especially if you wanted to be a surgeon.

Her reason for wanting us out of the way was twofold; to avoid being too close to the sterile field and to allow for room for us to faint as most students and residents did when it was their first surgery. Some people fainted for several surgeries. We were always instructed to make sure we ate lunch (yes, we had to be reminded as medical students sometimes), but in reality, some people fainted anyways at the sight of blood or bodily fluids. By us standing all the way back against the wall, this ensured that if we fainted, we wouldn't fall over onto the sterile surgical field. There were also chairs for us and we were told to sit down if we felt dizzy or lightheaded, a sign that we may be about to lose consciousness.

The surgery was for an incision and drainage procedure for an abscess on a man's butt. It was quite large and looked painful. The only thing that made me let out a tiny scream inside was the sight of his penis. Although I knew that he was going to be naked, I wasn't expecting him to be maneuvered in a way that his penis would fall out from under the drape and hang off the table. I felt like I wasn't supposed to be seeing his penis and I cringed a little. This man was my dad's age, a middle aged Black man and it felt wrong that I had full sight of his nakedness. Also, I couldn't see the operative field as well because they were working on his backside while I had full view of his front.

"Incision," one surgeon announced and within seconds of the announcement, a thick, foul smelling pus mixed with blood shot up in the air. Oh shit! That was a lot of pus in there. They continued to work on the abscess. It was large and they had vocalized that there were multiple smaller compartments they were trying to break up in efforts of draining all of the infected fluid. Despite not supposed to be interrupting during surgery, I asked to move. I couldn't see the action anymore. I also felt uncomfortable facing this man's penis that was dangling off the side of the bed in fetal position.

"Umm, excuse me?" I spoke up, "Excuse me, I cannot see what you guys are doing over there. Can I please come around to the other wall? I promise I won't touch anything." The two surgeons exchanged looks of surprise and approval and signaled for me to come on over to the other side of the room. I looked at my partner who came in the OR with me to see if they were going to come too. I realized they were sitting down and not looking well at all. I guess it was a good thing they gave us chairs. They must be used to us students needing a chair. I walked to the other side by myself and was able to watch the remainder of the surgery.

I felt pure bliss. This was hands down the best experience of the day and undoubtedly the best experience of the entire program. I remember sharing with Deonna about my day and how I got to wear scrubs and go into a surgery. She explained that she had only seen a dog get surgery. I was glad I wasn't in her group. Brianna was the coolest resident ever and had it not been for her advocating for me to go into a surgery, I would have likely never entered an operating room until I was a medical student. The remainder of the trip was phenomenal and every day, I was submerged in the curriculum so much that I didn't want the day to be over.

I called my parents every day as they had ordered me to do before I left. They were so happy I was having such a good time and loved hearing about my stories. My experience with NYLF at Emory played a pivotal role on my path of becoming a doctor. It solidified my lifelong dream and inspired me to enroll into the medical academy for my junior and senior years of high school. I truly think that my first O.R. experience confirmed that I belonged in the operating room and was a natural. Even at the age of 15, I wasn't grossed out, scared, or bored in surgery. I wanted to see more and I wanted to do more. I had always been told I was great with my hands, and this was one way to surely use my innate dexterity for the greater good. I will never forget that experience, and to this day, I am so very thankful for my parents, my grandmother, my uncle, and my grandpa for granting me that opportunity, as it truly propelled me forward in my journey of becoming a doctor.

Affirmation to recite: *I will capitalize on every opportunity that aids in identifying my purpose and calling. I understand the importance of opportunities and mentorship in achieving success and I want to make sure that I don't miss out on my blessing.*

Question: *Can you recall an experience or moment in your life when you decided on your career path? Are you still working in that field? Why or why not?*

CHAPTER 4

Decisions, Decisions

"Whatever we believe about ourselves and our ability comes true for us."

—Susan L. Taylor

As a girl who started off with very few friends who looked like me, to then being at a school district that had transformed to about 95% African American, most of my friends in middle and high school were Black. We shared many more commonalities that were lacking before. While I received an occasional "side eye" or smart comment about "talking White", for the most part, I was in a place that I felt very comfortable. As the end of high school neared, I longed for this feeling to continue. I wanted to be in a place where everyone looked like me, was raised similar to me, etc. I had been dancing my whole life (now at a majority Black dance school) and I wanted to continue that in college.

From watching TV, it appeared the experience I wanted would be best attained if I attended a historically Black College or University (HBCU). I began researching some of the different HBCUs. I even attended a "Black College

Tour" to learn more about various colleges that I did not know much about down south and the important history behind HBCUs. My grandfather was a professor at Florida Agricultural and Mechanical University (FAMU) and my Uncle Steve was a graduate of FAMU and Morgan State. Besides those schools, I did not know much about any others beside Howard University.

After the tour, and my self-guided research, I had decided that I would apply to Spelman College, Howard University, and Hampton University with Hampton being my number one choice. I felt obligated to apply to Michigan and Michigan State. They were two in-state schools, with great academic profiles and they would be my "back up plan".

I grew up watching Michigan sports, as my father and two uncles all attended the University of Michigan. I was bred a wolverine since birth. I even had the classic Starter Wolverines winter coat, spring jacket, ear muffs, and hat. But who wants to go to Michigan? Are there Black people in Ann Arbor? Will they have an awesome band and hip hop dance team? From my experience watching the cheerleaders on television, there was always one on the team, no more, no less. Of course, academics were stellar at Michigan, but I was smart and I knew I could excel anywhere. I just wanted to be around "my people". God forbid I go back to being a minority again and dealing with racism and the "fitting in" conundrum, as I did in my childhood.

As focused as I was on the negative aspects of why I did not want to go to Michigan, I had to tap into my inner mature aspiring doctor self for a moment. I knew I wanted to be a doctor and medical school was my goal immediately following college. I wanted to attend a school that would have the resources, academics, and support to be able to help get me there. I did not have any medical doctors in my family, so I knew that I would need to attend a school with the resources to be able to assist me in getting there. For that reason and that reason alone, Michigan did not seem too bad at all. Well, besides the fact that I enjoyed Michigan Football and attending games would be another bonus. This was a hard decision, but I cast a wide net and would deal with this decision later on after applying.

When deciding on what college to attend, I was glad that I cast a wide net. It is easy to limit oneself based on rumors, self-confidence, or your comfort zone. College is a time that you really mature into your adult self so it is important to choose a school where you can see growth and maturity in your future. One common mistake I see many people make is picking a college based on his/her friends. Everyone's needs and career interests are different so this is the time to branch out of that comfort zone that high school had many of us nestled in. If you're like most students, you're undecided on a major until midway through college anyways, so picking a school that has a variety of different programs for you to choose from is beneficial. Most importantly, choose a school where you feel at home, have a good support system nearby, and some fun extracurricular activities. Let's face it, you're not going to spend four years at college with your nose in the books everyday. Have fun! Let your hair down.

I remember speaking to mentors and teachers at my school about deciding what college I was going to attend. My guidance counselor as well as teachers all felt that I was an excellent student and would excel wherever I went and wrote letters of recommendation to support that sentiment. At this point in my life, I had always performed exceptionally well in school, was confident in my potential, and was surrounded by people who believed in me. My parents were adamant about pushing my brother and me, and to not place limitations on our potential. I didn't know what it felt like to not have support at home nor being told that I couldn't achieve whatever it was I wanted to do. This was very different from both of my parents' experience.

My mother is from Buffalo, New York. When they were in elementary school, her parents, my grandparents, moved out of the predominantly Black neighborhood to a suburb that allegedly had better schools. Little did my mother and uncle Steve know at the time, that it would mean they would be one of the only few Black families in the neighborhood, and the first two Black students at their school. This was a culture shock to them after moving from a predominantly Black area of Buffalo prior to that. It was an adjustment to them and being that this was in the 1960s, there was quite a bit of racism and taunting that came along for the ride.

My mom hated her school so much that she wanted to graduate early to move on to college. In part, this was shortly after my grandparents had divorced and I am sure that played a role, but also she didn't feel like she fit in there. When she went to the guidance counselor for advice about applying to college, she was met with resistance. The counselor told my mother that with her natural beauty, thin figure, and tall stature she would be better off pursuing a career in modeling. If she didn't want to be a model, the counselor suggested trade school would be a great alternative. Luckily, my mom had two parents that were supportive of her dreams of going to college, as they were both college educated themselves, and she did not let that deter her from applying.

Not only did she get accepted to multiple colleges, she received academic scholarships as well. She ended up attending the University of Buffalo after finishing high school in 3 years. My mom also finished college with a bachelor's degree in 3 years as well. Hearing stories about my mom when she was younger was no surprise to me. She still has that same drive and ambition with everything she sets out to do. She has always scolded me for being too hard on myself and pushing my limits to unreasonable thresholds and to the harshest critique, but she has always been the exact same way. She made it a point to make sure that Melvin and I knew that we could do anything we wanted to do and that college was not an option for us. She took education very seriously and made sure we understood the value of it at an early age.

My father is from Romulus, which was a rural town outside of Detroit, and grew up just down the street from the

Detroit airport. His upbringing was very different from my mother's. His parents owned quite a bit of land, farms filled with hogs, chickens—you name it. He and his two brothers, Michael and Aaron, grew up driving tractors, working in the yard, and hunted regularly with their dad. Their household was very traditional with my grandma staying home and caring for the kids and the household and cooking hot meals three times a day. My grandma didn't even own a microwave until I was in college! My Granddad worked at Ford Motor Company for decades. He and my grandma had moved to the Detroit area from Arkansas and Alabama as a part of the "The Great Migration".

The Great Migration, from 1916 to 1970, one of the largest internal migrations in the history of the United States, was a mass movement of about five million southern African-Americans that headed north or west in search of jobs, better education, and less racism. Since the emancipation of slavery, the economy and structure in the south allowed for very little opportunities of growth for Blacks as well as the harsh discrimination and upheld Jim Crow laws in the south. After World War I, there were many factories in the north that had jobs for Blacks to work in and this was a much better lifestyle and earning potential for them. Many Blacks who migrated to Detroit went to work for Ford Motor Company, which, at that time, was the largest employer of Blacks in the city. Ford Motor company was known for paying Black workers and White workers equal pay for equal work which was unheard of back then. This presented an attractive opportunity for many southern Blacks, including my granddad.

Having a father like my granddad, it was impossible for my dad and uncles to not know what hard work was, even at a young age. Although neither of their parents had attended school beyond eighth grade, they held their children to the highest standard after making sure they provided them an environment to support that feat. My dad rarely got in trouble in school because he knew the consequences he would have to face when his father got home if he acted up. Being the oldest of three boys, he had to set the example for his brothers to follow, as his parents expected of him.

My dad knew that he wanted to be an architect since he was in the eighth grade and he knew that he would do just that one day. When he came toward the completion of high school, he met with his guidance counselor which was a requirement to get an application for college. He knew that his parents didn't have the money to send him to college out of state and there were only a few architecture schools in the state of Michigan at the time. Growing up watching Michigan sports and looking into their architecture program, he really wanted to attend the University of Michigan. They had a six-year program that once you were accepted, you continued through the six years to obtain a bachelor's and master's degree. This is the program he was passionate about getting accepted into. When he asked for the application from the counselor, the counselor looked my dad in the eyes in laughed.

"Melvin, you won't be accepted into a school like the University of Michigan, so I will not let you waste your time. Have you considered trade school?" the counselor asked my dad.

"I want to attend the University of Michigan's school of architecture and I have great grades. If they are going to turn me down, I would rather hear it from them," my dad shot back.

"I'm sorry I cannot support this and will not be giving you the application," the counselor ended the conversation. My dad did not feel it was worth going back and forth because he had heard from multiple other students that looked like him that they received the same response. He didn't understand why the counselor cared so much about him applying. If he got rejected, that was on him, but he could not live with himself NOT trying. My dad was driven as well and when he wanted something, he wouldn't accept no as an answer. Of course, if Michigan sent him a rejection letter, he would have to accept that, but why was the counselor not even allowing him to apply to Michigan? Why was he telling all the other Black students the same thing? He could have just given up but that wasn't who my dad was or is even today.

My dad pulled out the yellow pages directory and sent a letter to the University of Michigan admissions office asking for an application. For my younger readers, the yellow pages was a huge phone book with numbers and addresses to companies and other institutions in a pretty widespread radius from where you lived. This was frequently circulated and dropped off in your driveway or at your doorstep just like the newspaper. This was also pre-internet days so he couldn't just navigate to their website and apply online or request an application. He had to send a letter via snail mail. He included in his letter why he wanted to attend Michigan and what program he wanted to matriculate in. A few weeks later, he received an application in the mail. Excited and motivated by this small gesture, my dad completed the application and mailed it in. Not only was he accepted, but he received a full scholarship to attend. He couldn't wait to share that with the counselor who had refused to give him one of the many blank applications he had a pile of sitting behind his desk!

Knowing what my parents had to go through to even be able to apply to college made me have an appreciation for the application process. I didn't have any counselors withholding applications from me or telling me I should consider trade school when I made it clear that I wanted to be a doctor. Everyone at my school was supportive of my dreams, as was my family. They truly believed that I would one day become a doctor and that belief made me believe in myself even more. Everyone does not always have a great support system, and sometimes believing in oneself can be enough to propel you toward your dream. But I will say, it was the support system for me. That's what kept me motivated.

I stand by this advice to this day: do not choose a college based off your friends. As we entered junior and senior year, we had all received letters and applications from different schools in and out of state. Some were sent in mass mailings to everyone in certain zip codes and others were targeted based on grade point average (GPA), athletic accolades, or other activities that made applicants appear more favorable. I felt the same way about college brochures then as I do about spam emails now. I was sick of them! Every day, a new college or two or ten was sending brochures on why their school was the best. My best friend Deonna had received a brochure from Saginaw Valley, an in-state public school about an hour away from home and she fell in love. She really wanted to go there or to Michigan. Being that she was 16 years old, with a license and a car, she suggested that our "BTD crew" (Brittany, Tamika, Deonna) took a mini road trip up there to tour the school. Brittany and I were down for a fun girls' trip especially at that age. We packed up Deonna's brand new Black Kia Rio and headed up to Saginaw, Michigan.

This was not the first college campus tour for any of us. Deonna and I had participated in the NYLF program the summer prior at Emory University in Atlanta. All three of us had also gone on a Black college tour. They went on one through Brittany's church, Hartford Memorial. As much as I wanted to attend the tour with them, the HBCUs I was interested in at that time: Howard, Hampton, Xavier, and Spelman weren't included in their route. Although I kept my parents' pockets empty with all my activities I explored, I didn't believe in wasting their money. I knew that the trip would just be a good time with my girls but really not give me any additional value from touring schools that I wanted to apply to. I decided to go on a Black college tour the same year, but I went with a different church. I was a little hesitant because I didn't have any close friends on that trip, but I knew a few people going and I was always a social butterfly and loved meeting new people from all over. That was the first decision that I made for myself regarding college that was not centered around my friends.

Saginaw Valley's campus was nice! It was much different than the HBCUs I had visited previously, but I expected that. Many of these schools that lacked diversity always had the most diverse pictures on the brochures they sent to the house, but when you got to the campus, you realized that you would be a part of the minority there. I noticed the same thing I had noticed at the University of Michigan's campus—it seemed pretty segregated. Black students sat with Black students. White students sat with White students. Asian students sat with Asian students, and so forth. I'm sure it wasn't formally designed to be that segregated, but it was something that I noticed at all of these non HBCU colleges, frequently referred to as PWIs, or primarily white institutions.

After seeing the campus, the three of us reflected how fun it would be if we all went to college together or at least very close nearby so we could party together and continue hanging out as we had since the seventh grade. I loved my BFFs and that idea sounded dope!

"Ok, so let's grab the applications while we are up here and we can all apply as soon as we get back home!" Deonna suggested.

"Sounds like a decent plan. I'm down!" Brittany agreed. I kept quiet because deep down I knew I really had no intention of attending the school. They both followed suit and turned their application in and received acceptance letters later that fall.

Why couldn't I just say that I didn't want to apply there? The truth is I felt bad. We had always been BTD and longed for the opportunity to go to college together and spend time with each other. Brittany was also considering Northwood, which was a school about twenty minutes away. She had received information in the mail and had a few older students from high school that attended there and loved it. She was in the business academy in high school and wanted to pursue a career in business or marketing. Northwood had an excellent business program.

I didn't have a passion or reason for attending either school. If I stayed in state, I was going to go to the most competitive school there was, and that was the University of Michigan in Ann Arbor. It was the top public university in the entire country right there, 45 minutes from home. I had taken it for granted but deep down I knew that Michigan was an excellent school and it would be cool to follow in my father's footsteps. My biggest concern was about my social life and the lack of diversity I noticed on their campus.

Saginaw and Northwood were lacking in those areas too. I worked my butt off to maintain a great academic profile, involvement in community service and leadership activities, all to get into the best college I could, so why am I going to forfeit that for my friends?

Surely, we would still see each other and party on the weekends. Maybe not every weekend, but I am sure we would take turns visiting one another if I stayed in state. I never turned the application in to either school.

With my heart full of optimism, I sent off my college applications to Spelman, Howard, Hampton, University of Michigan and Michigan State. Well technically, for Michigan State, they performed onsite interviews at my high school. If you had above a certain GPA, they would grant you an onsite interview where they would set up a date and call you to the counseling office. At the end of the interview, they would hand you an acceptance letter.

So at that time, I had already received an acceptance letter to Michigan State. I received acceptance letters from the other four schools with full scholarship offers from every school I applied to, including Michigan State. Although it did not help me narrow anything down, it was something I was extremely proud of. To be perfectly honest, I was not surprised that I got into all five schools; my mentors and teachers had gassed me up enough that I knew I would likely get in. I certainly did not think I was going to receive a full tuition scholarship for four years from every school though. That took the cake.

At that point, where every school was offering me the same thing, how was I supposed to narrow down my decision? I had no desire to attend Michigan or Michigan State; they were my back up plans. I will admit though, after receiving a full scholarship, I had to rethink my rash decision of counting those schools out. If I stayed in state and chose not to go to an HBCU, I would definitely attend Michigan over Michigan State. It was a better school, and I grew up with maize and blue in my blood, why would I ever take a second look at a less competitive school. (Ok, that was a mini inter-school rivalry jab, but hey, I am a wolverine, through and through!)

It took a lot of self-reflection, discussions with teachers, friends, and most importantly, my parents to help me make a final decision. When I was seconds away from choosing Hampton University to attend, I ended up choosing the University of Michigan. This was a top public institution, right in our backyard essentially, and could potentially offer me the resources to be able to get to medical school. Not that I felt that Hampton would not get me there, but I felt I needed to jump onto this opportunity to attend the top public university in the country at the time and have the luxury of being only 45 minutes away from home.

I honestly felt this was the best decision for my career, but not for my social life as I recall myself envisioning at the tender age of 16 when I accepted Michigan's full ride offer. This was a very mature decision that I still pat myself on the back for to this day. I chose the school that was best for my academics and career rather than the one I would feel more comfortable at, with awesome parties, Greek life, etc.

> ***Affirmation to recite:*** *I will make decisions for myself. Although some decisions may be influenced by others, I will be sure to consider myself first.*
>
> **Question:** *When have you made a major decision for someone else and regretted it?*

Part II

The Caterpillar (College)

CHAPTER 5

Stay Mad, Abby!

"You can't be a minority in this society without having someone express disapproval about affirmative action."

—Sonia Sotomayor

The University of Michigan campus in Ann Arbor is still one of the most beautiful college campuses I have ever been on. Walking on campus for the first time as an enrolled student felt amazing. I remember feeling overwhelmed for the first couple of weeks because everything was spread out, I frequently got lost and I had to take the bus to get around campus and that was an adjustment. This was all very new to me, as it was for most college freshmen.

Despite the feeling of being overwhelmed, I frequently stopped on the DIAG, took a look around and was proud of myself for getting there. The DIAG was our large open courtyard space that many of the major central campus buildings and libraries open up to. Frequently this was a social gathering spot, studying spot, and an area to have events and fundraisers. This is the one of the busiest places on central campus and you had the best chance at running into almost everyone at some point during the day.

Central campus was huge, with not only academic buildings, but also with bars, restaurants, boutiques, and shops situated throughout our campus. It was not uncommon for students to visit some of the local merchants during long two to three-hour breaks between classes. My roommate Nita and I frequented these local shops in between classes because our dorm room was on North campus; which was a fifteen-minute bus ride away. By the time we waited at the bus stop, took the bus up to north campus, got off and walked to our dorm, and the time to repeat the steps in reverse order to get to class, many times it was just easier to hang around campus. This was also our opportunity to meet other students, participate in local events or fundraisers and try to really soak up the "college experience".

Being at a top institution with this large, beautiful campus and tons of extracurricular activities, what else could a student ask for, right? Eh... not so much.

Aside from the wonderful things mentioned and the exhilarating "football Saturdays" in Ann Arbor, and the awesome hip hop dance team we had joined, we actually pretty much hated Michigan during our first year. Where was the exaggerated amount of diversity that was expressed on the brochures and pamphlets they sent to the house? Was there a secret hidden place where all the minorities hung out? Nita and I frequently planned out how we should transfer to another school together because this was not going to work out for us. Every week there seemed to be more ammunition to support why we did not belong there.

Most of my classes, I was the only Black person and if I was lucky, maybe one other would join me. This was significantly different from my high school. It did not bother me much being the minority; what bothered me most were the interactions that frequently happened as a result. As a student who had always absolutely loved school and learning, I was always volunteering in class, asking questions and engaged especially in math and science classes as they were my favorite subjects.

I will never forget my calculus class freshman year. Part of our curriculum was team homework assignments. We would get together outside the classroom to do the homework, turn it in for a group grade, and in class would discuss the problems and work them out together on the board.

Our calculus group met in front of the undergraduate library (students referred to it as "The UGLi") and once everyone had arrived we headed to the back to find a table to do our homework assignments. Each group member had worked out the problems individually and came together to compile our answers as a group. Ben showed his math problems to the group. Quick glance from other team members with a confirmatory nod. Sarah went on to share her assigned problems. She was met with the same affirmation by the group. Next, it was my turn to share my answers.

"Let me see that, Tamika. I want to review it," Ben stated, then began meticulously reviewing what I had done. *Is he serious?* I stayed silent.

"Ben, which problems did Tamika do? I want to work them out while you're looking at that," Sarah interjected.

"Well guys, I did problems one through four. Here is my notebook so you can see how I arrived at my answers," I explained. It was like my voice was nonexistent. Not one of the group members looked up to see what I was showing them in my notebook. This became a weekly ritual and I frequently took a more passive approach. I did not want to be the aggressive Black girl in the group shouting that my answer was correct. I mean... but it *was* though. I definitely spent a lot of time working on my answers as did everyone else. I was confident with my answers, just like everyone else in the group was. I am not saying that I never made mistakes, but I did not understand why my work was always reviewed with this level of scrutiny.

Math was one of my stronger subjects and I caught on pretty fast. Not to mention that I had taken Advanced Placement (AP) Calculus in high school. Yet here we are spending an additional forty minutes "checking my work". Why weren't other team members' work being reviewed, questioned, and checked? After noticing the pattern, I became so frustrated and annoyed that I began dreading our team homework meetings. Might I add, my answers always "checked out" to be correct. Surprise, surprise.

I was not used to people not listening to me. In high school, many peers accepted each others' input, as we recognized we were all intelligent and could help each other get to the goal. But this was different. I could not help but to think it had something to do with the fact that I was the Black girl in the group. This made for very frustrating group work in this class.

One day I will likely never forget, I was sitting in this same calculus class reviewing the team homework problems as a class. There was a math problem my teacher was working out on the board and asking students for input. Everyone was giving answers, and instead of him stating if they were right or wrong, he kept asking for other students input before he would share the answer with us. For the first time in my life, I did not feel comfortable raising my hand, or taking a chance on being wrong. I felt like all eyes were on me and I did not want to get the answer wrong publicly so I kept my hand down. I actually felt pretty confident about my answer based on what he had just taught us the week prior but there was no way I was going to raise my hand at that moment. After all, what if I was wrong?

I could not escape participating that day, because my professor called on me. I remember thinking to myself, *I did not raise my hand! Why would you call on the one person not raising her hand? Is he picking on me because I am Black?* I hesitantly went to the board, worked up the problem with the answer then sat back in my seat.

Some of the other students were snickering and whispering things such as "That is wrong! Oh my gosh, how embarrassing. What's wrong with her?" My teacher began asking students why this was wrong and I thought to myself, *what is he doing? I am totally dropping this class today! He did not do this with any of the other students. He always seemed so nice during his office hours! Why would he embarrass me like this?*

Students continued laughing and snickering at my "wrong answer" and the feeling I was trying to avoid came over me all at once. I purposely did not raise my hand because I did not want to be the "dumb Black girl" in the class if I got the answer wrong, yet here I am, feeling like the "dumb Black girl". I have never felt so little in my life. I was holding back tears sitting in a class full of laughter.

My teacher looked over at me and smiled. Why was he smiling? Was he happy that he made me feel this way? I am absolutely dropping this course after class. I would have to find another section because I needed this course as a pre-requisite for applying to medical school. My teacher stood at the front of the room and stated, "Tamika was the only correct answer!" He then went on to explain why my answer was correct and pointed to the work that I had written on the board. No wonder he was smiling. Maybe he wasn't so bad after all. Even in that moment of being right, I still did not feel much better. A couple of my classmates whom I always sat with, gave me a fist bump for getting the answer right. I still did not feel any better. I walked out of class that day still fighting back my tears.

My professor asked me to meet him in his office after class. When I went to talk to him, the tears came rushing out. He comforted me in that moment and explained how disappointed he was in the class for their behavior today. He also exclaimed how proud of me he was and that I should never feel "dumb" or "incompetent" because of other people's remarks or laughter. "Tamika, I called on you because I knew you would know the right answer. I did not call on you to humiliate you. I wanted you to work the problem out on the board because I knew you had the answer. You didn't raise your hand but you knew the answer!"

I explained to him that I always felt inferior, classmates always rechecked my team homework answers and that I overall was struggling with the transition to a huge institution where I was the minority. It's funny because I never once mentioned that I was planning to drop the class, yet he suggested that option to me. He explained that I would probably excel better in a different class with a different group of students who may not behave this way. He also explained that he noticed my interactions with other students previously and he could definitely see why I felt so uncomfortable. At that moment, my pride would not let me succumb to my inner feelings.

I wiped my tears and told him, "I am not dropping the class because of this silly behavior. I will see you in class next week! Thanks for the pep talk!" And just like that, I had made up my mind to stay in that class and ignore any future negativity.

With much surprise on his face, he ended our meeting with a smile and a handshake. Although I was minutes from dropping the course, when it was suggested to me I looked at it from a completely different angle. I could not let this deter me from my goals. I loved my teacher, I was learning a lot, and I just had to be tougher and keep my eyes on the prize. This class would be over in just a few months, and my discomfort being a minority at Michigan would continue for years. Never would I imagine that this one incident would shape my outlook and play such a pivotal role in my approach to similar situations to come later in life.

As a firm believer of God ordained paths, I knew that it was no coincidence that the events that took place when I was in Ann Arbor happened when I was there. The calculus incident was one of many more to come and I needed that to happen in order to help me navigate other future incidents smoothly.

As mentioned before, the DIAG was our large open space where many students crossed walking to class, hung out in between classes, and where events would take place. One day after class, when I was walking from Angel Hall (on the west side of the DIAG) to the North Campus bus stop (Northeast side of the DIAG), I saw a large crowd around a stage with a person shouting into a bullhorn. The thing that stood out the most to me was that the crowd were students from elementary up to college age. These were students that had been bussed from the Metro Detroit Area. I had to move quickly so I could catch the next bus to north campus in time for a meeting. I tapped one of the college students from the periphery of the crowd to ask what was going on. She told me, "They are here protesting for affirmative action." Reverend Al Sharpton had attended the event and led the rally of over 1000 attendees in protest of the recent racial climates.

To give you some reference, I attended Michigan from 2005 to 2009, right through the thick of the affirmative action debates and protests. Michigan had historically used a 150-point system for admission to the university. Minorities would receive an additional 20 points in this system. In June 2003, just two years before I matriculated at the University of Michigan, the ruling in the Supreme court case, Gratz v. Bollinger was that this 20-point "advantage" for minorities was unconstitutional. Some argued that a perfect SAT score was only worth 12 points in this system, but race alone was worth a "whopping 20 points". Needless to say, the admission policy was changed as a result. Student groups on campus and local leaders and activists were infuriated by this decision.

I got on the Bursley-Baits Bus (bus to north campus dorms) with a million thoughts on my mind about the protest, the affirmative action cases, and the overall racial climate on campus. I sat quietly on the bus when another student, a Caucasian male, started a conversation with me about the protest. The bus was packed that time of day-students standing, sitting, and packed like sardines trying to get back to their respective dorms after a long day of classes. *Why was he picking my brain about this right now?*

"Hey did you see all those students on the DIAG protesting?" he probed while standing in the aisle next to my seat.

I looked up at him and responded, "Yes of course."

Another student chimed in, "What are they even protesting? They have been out there all day!"

The conversation starter responded quickly, "They are protesting the ban on affirmative action. This is so ridiculous. I mean, I am not racist or anything but I just want everything to be equal. You know? It's not fair that y'all get into a top school like this just because you're Black. The rest of us have to work hard to get here, so why can't it be the same for y'all?"

I responded, "Well, for starters, we work hard to get here too. I graduated in the top 10% of my class and scored exceptionally well on my ACT—the same standardized exam that you took. Why would you assume that I am any less qualified than the next student?"

He continued probing, "Well how do you know if you got here because of merit or just because you're Black? You know they give 20 extra points to y'all for being Black!"

Another student questioned, "Wow, 20 points just for being Black?"

"I am familiar with the point system you're referring to. I know that I am here because of merit because that Supreme court case ruling was two years ago, in June 2003.

I am a freshman who was admitted after that ruling. Also, I am here on a full academic scholarship. You think I received that for being Black too?" I responded. *When was this bus ride going to be over?* Tensions were getting high and I could not ignore his ignorance. "Furthermore, to address your comment on equality. You say you want us all to have equal playing grounds for admission, right?" I continued.

"Yes. That's all I am saying. I am all for Blacks coming to my school, but only under the same exact admission criteria. Equal across the board. Now that's fair," he announced. Other students sitting near us nodded their heads in agreement. *Did he really just say "his school"? Wasn't it our school?*

"Our backgrounds are not equal, our history and resources are not equal. Our education in our school systems are not equal. But you somehow feel that the admission criteria for all should be equal? You think that the student who attended all 12 grades of school without a textbook, in a classroom with 40 other students, no money for private tutoring and preparation courses, working a part time job in high school to help feed their family, who still managed to get the same or damn near standardized test score and GPA shouldn't be looked at favorably when compared to the student from a top collegiate prep private school with a private tutor, a classroom with 20 students, textbooks for every class and not having to work after school?"

Silence.

"I cannot continue to have this conversation with you. Until you understand the minorities' plight in getting to these 'esteemed universities', you will never understand that without affirmative action, many of us wouldn't be afforded the same opportunities that we deserve," I snapped back.

The bus pulled up to the curb at Bursley Hall. I grabbed my bookbag and hopped off the bus. I had only been a college student at Michigan for a couple months and I was not feeling this at all.

Little did I know, the affirmative action conversation would be one that would continue for the rest of my college career and beyond. The following year, some friends and I participated in events and rallies prior to the election. Proposal 2 was a proposal to ban affirmative action for public education, employees and contracting in the state of Michigan. Supporters of this ban were spreading the word that "Prop 2 is about affirmative action", in hopes that uninformed minority voters would infer that this proposal was in favor of affirmative action and vote yes. In actuality, although it was in fact "about affirmative action", it was a ban on affirmative action. Our goal with Black Student Union, NAACP, and other student groups on campus was to inform voters that we want to vote "No" on Prop 2. Prop 2 would ban affirmative action in the state of Michigan and would be detrimental to the minority enrollment not only at our school, but all institutions across the state.

The Michigan electorate approved Proposal 2 on November 7th, 2006. Six years later, in 2012, the appeals court threw out this ban, only to have it upheld again in April 2014. As a result, this back and forth has become a central political conversation to this day.

In 2008, a student at the University of Texas (UT), Abigail Fisher, sued the university for declined admission. The school uses affirmative action to assist in minority enrollment and Abigail argued that this was not fair. In July 2014, the US Supreme Court ruled that the university could continue using race as a factor in admissions in effort to bring more diversity to the university. At that time, UT considered applicants based on an Academic Index (AI) and Personal Achievement Index (PAI). These consider class rank, standardized test scores, socioeconomic status, and race. It was released that Abigail had an AI of 3.1 and PAI of less than 6. UT stated that due to the steep competition in 2008, even if she had received a perfect PAI score of 6, with her "average" AI score of 3.1, she still would not have been admitted. The statement implied that her grades were "just not good enough".

My esteemed reader, if you're an avid social media junkie, you may remember the hashtag #staymadabby. This was a hashtag born as a result of that ruling. Minorities were posting pictures of collegiate acceptances and accolades in addition to quotes while using the tag #staymadabby. This led to a viral movement to spread awareness of the need for affirmative action, and that those who are granted admission through affirmative action were just as qualified and going on to win national awards, matriculate in top graduate schools, and attain competitive jobs in various industries.

Due to the ongoing affirmative action controversy I experienced on campus when I was a student—I could go on all day about affirmative action, but I have to move on... the bottom line is that affirmative action is necessary. It is not unfair. An "equal playing ground" in lieu of hundreds of years of inequities historically that are still present to this very day is an absurd request. We can table this discussion though. You either feel me, or you don't.

Affirmation to recite: *I deserve to be here just as much as the person next to me.*

Question: *When was a time that someone else's doubts of you impacted how you view yourself? Why did it impact you? Would it still impact you today?*

CHAPTER 6

Does Success Look Like Me?

"I have learned not to allow rejection to move me."

—Cicely Tyson

Upon enrollment at Michigan, each student is assigned an advisor. This person is your go-to-person for information about programs, declaring a major, future career goals, etc. This was a huge university but being assigned an advisor helped students stay on the right track for graduation and to help students feel they had an ongoing resource to go to throughout your time at the school. For this reason, your advisor would stay your advisor throughout your four years there. We were instructed to meet with our advisors regularly throughout the year.

My first meeting with my advisor was, in fact, my last. She was very pleasant and easy to talk to. During our meeting she asked what my career goals were. She assured me, "Tamika, it's ok if you are unsure because it is common for students to not know for the first couple years they are exploring."

I explained that this was not the case for me. "I want to be a pediatrician!" I got a blank stare.

"A doctor? Well we do not have a structured pre-medicine program. Students typically declare a subject specific major and take all the pre-requisites for medical school and apply if the time comes." *Did she just say if? I thought I made it clear that my mind was set on becoming a doctor.* She then went on to explain, "Most students start off with a pre-med or pre-law intention but most students never actually go to medical school or law school." *Ok, the course load is competitive. Got it.* I guess she observed that I was not fully grasping her subtleties, because she continued on.

"Tamika, most of us minorities do not become doctors or even get into medical school. It is a very difficult path that can be very discouraging when we do not get in. What typically happens is that students enroll in all the hard science pre-med courses, do not do very well, then it ends up pulling your GPA down. When you don't get into medical school and need to go another route, your GPA will have suffered from all the science courses. It is very difficult to maintain a high GPA with that course load."

I responded, "Well I want to be a doctor. I want to start taking my biology and chemistry courses."

My advisor objected, "My job is to advise you and this is not a good route to take. You all usually do better in business. Have you thought about applying to the business school here? We have one of the top business schools in the country. During your first two years, you should 'explore' and take courses in different areas before you decide to take science classes. Do you have any interest in business or marketing? What about communications?"

My naïve freshman self entered a mental fog. Well, in high school, I was in a marketing organization called DECA. We competed on various business topics and I was pretty good at it. I think I could do well in marketing. Maybe she was right. I heard from several peers that the organic chemistry courses here are crazy hard. I would hate to pull my GPA down just to get a rejection from medical school. Maybe I should stick to something I know I am good at.

After pondering awhile, I responded, "Ok, that sounds like a good plan. I won't enroll in any science classes for now. Thank you!" *I needed to think further about the business school, but what I did know was that I was thankful to have someone help me. I could have just ruined my GPA if it wasn't for my advisor.*

Pause. Typing the thoughts that went through my head at that time still infuriate me to this day even as an accomplished physician. How could I have been that stupid to let this lady change my whole lifelong dream in a thirty-minute conversation? Needless to say, I ended up enrolling in the pre-requisites for the business school. This meant I had to take Microeconomics.

About thirty minutes into the first microeconomics lecture about supply and demand curve basics, I remember thinking to myself "I am so glad I listened to my advisor. This is easy." The class got increasingly boring from that day on, and I was frequently fighting off sleep. It was much to my surprise that I totally bombed my first exam. To keep it simple, what I thought made sense, apparently made no sense at all. I engaged in countless amounts of tutoring sessions, office hours with the professor, and studying in the library that semester to achieve my God given grade of a C. Yes, Tamika Cross got her first C, and I worked hard for it!

Fast forward to another semester of prerequisites for the business school (no, I still had not learned my lesson that that was not my calling). I applied to the business school at the end of my first year and received my first rejection letter in my life. I was embarrassed and I remember only sharing this with one of my good childhood friends, Marcus, and maybe my roommate. Marcus was always business savvy and this was definitely his calling, not mine. He was one of the few people that even knew that I had applied, so I felt it was only natural to share with him my rejection and devastation. So let's take a step back, by listening to the advisor, I allowed her to deter me from my lifelong dream, to focus on a path that I knew was not my calling, in efforts of protecting my GPA and scholarship. Only to earn my first C and rejection letter to the business school.

The famous quote goes "when life gives you lemons, make lemonade" and that resonated with me deeply as a result of my first year. I was crushed by my C and rejection letter. I saw it as a failure. I was not a C student. I secretly considered dropping out because I was convinced Michigan was too hard for me and I did not belong there. I'm glad I got my act together quickly and didn't sulk in self-pity for too long. Many of us have a tendency of doing that. It's not productive. God watched me make this huge mistake in denying my calling to become a physician and this "rejection" was necessary for Him to get me back on track in becoming a doctor. I went through a series of emotions and pep talks with myself and my parents. As a result, I made a humbling call to one of my childhood friends, Chi, who was also pre-med at the University of Michigan. I asked him if he still wanted to be a doctor. After he assured me that his plans were still on track, I began asking him when was he going to start taking pre-med classes. He responded with surprise.

"Umm, I am taking my third science class this semester. You know we have to apply for medical school at the end of our junior year if you do not take a year off. There are a lot of classes to take in a short period of time," Chi replied.

I don't remember if I ever told him about my recent rejection to the business school that month. I probably didn't. I was embarrassed that I had even applied to the school and even more embarrassed that I did not get in. I had known Chi since 4th grade and we had shared our mutual affinity for medicine and were in the medical academy in high school together. Most of our AP science classes, we had taken together as well. My pride at that age probably would have never allowed me to tell him that I had fallen victim to a certain piece of advice about not applying for medical school. I was proud that he had kept at it. I needed to play catch up. An entire year had gone by and I had not taken a single science class. Chi, if you're reading this, thank you. He probably does not even remember this conversation, as it was insignificant to him, but it goes to show how one small conversation can make such a huge impact in someone else's life.

Although I was excited about my summer vacation approaching and spending it with all my friends that would be home from college, I knew I needed to play catch up if I wanted to complete the courses that would be tested on the MCAT (medical college admissions test). My scholarship only covered classes during fall and winter semesters. It did not cover summer school. I knew I needed to take classes in the summer if I wanted to finish on time. The cost did not deter my parents. They had banked on the fact that my schooling was free and probably budgeted for that as well. So I was super appreciative that they understood I had made a huge mistake and were willing to help me pay for summer school. That summer, I enrolled in summer classes at Oakland Community College.

The catch up continued throughout my sophomore year as well. When the summer of 2007 came up, I knew I needed another summer of classes to catch up. The classes were relatively inexpensive at the community college so I figured I would pay and plan for another summer filled with classes. I was still working my part time job at Footlocker and a part time job on campus so I would be able to pay for it. At that point I was involved in a handful of on-campus organizations and had met a lot of friends at school. I remember using my network to discuss my plan for summer school again. I am glad that I did.

My peer shared with me that after you have 60 college credits at Michigan, you cannot take classes at the community college anymore to count toward your major. I looked this rule up online to find out that this was true. That would have been tragic.

This information was a great save but it highlighted another issue. I needed summer school as I was still playing catch up, but it would have to be at Michigan where the courses were much more expensive than my community college budget, and that meant I couldn't go home for the summer again. My parents came to the rescue again. They again helped pay for my summer courses in 2007. I continued playing catch up for my remaining years in college. It was worth it though. I finished my degree in four years. My scholarship was for four years so this was absolutely necessary.

I spent a few years... ok maybe more than a few years... resenting my college advisor who sent me on this deviated path, discouraged me from becoming a physician, who cost me a C on my transcript, a rejection letter from the business school, three summers spent in school, and the tuition bill to accompany it. It took growth, maturity, meditation, and prayer for me to change my outlook on this situation. Although she advised me to drop my science courses, apply for the business school, and forget about becoming a doctor, her advice was just that. Advice. I did not have to take her advice. I could have stood my ground and stayed on course. It was my lifelong dream, not hers. It was my job to defend it. What is the point of having a dream if you are not willing to stand by it, defend it, climb obstacles, and work for it? This was necessary for me to go through to realize the importance of dreaming and the importance of perseverance. I never again let another soul convince me I was not going to accomplish anything I dreamed of accomplishing.

> ***Affirmation to recite:*** *Society's unrealistic dreams are attainable goals.*
>
> **Question:** *Can you recall a time when someone else's discouraging words deterred you from striving toward your dreams? Why did their words have that effect on you?*

CHAPTER 7

Hustle and Grind

"Everybody has a dream but not everybody has a grind."

—Eric Thomas

During the series of me playing catch up with my classes, I also had joined multiple on-campus organizations. One of the organizations was the Black Pre-Medical Association (BPMA) and it served as an excellent resource for us pre-med students. My friend Chanel informed me about this organization and I decided to join her. We were able to get matched with mentors who were medical students, residents, and attending physicians. During our meetings, we had talks about the process of becoming a doctor, what you need to consider for applications and interviews, etc. For other students who were like me, the first medical doctor in their family, we were really in the dark on the process of becoming a doctor.

This organization was a game changer for me and I made many long-lasting relationships as a result of BPMA. One of the programs we had was a shadowing program where we could shadow doctors in the field we were interested in going into. I expressed that I wanted to be a pediatrician so I was matched with a Pediatric Infectious Disease physician, Dr. Blackwood. By his agreement to allow me to shadow him, his role was to allow me to round with him and the team, and answer questions about the field. It is an understatement to say he exceeded his expectation by far and became a mentor of mine who I hold near and dear to my heart. Our initial meetings were intense...

At that point, I had taken several science courses and earned all As and Bs. I was pretty proud of myself. Even in my first Organic Chemistry, one of the hardest courses at Michigan, I had earned a B. I remember sitting in his office one day and him telling me that his goal was to get me to one day be his replacement. I did not believe him at the time, but now over ten years later looking back, I know he meant it. He asked me about my grades. Grades were not everything but they were important for getting into medical school, so he wanted to make sure I was on track. I remember smiling while sharing that I had all As and Bs. I was so proud of myself! He asked me what I received in Organic Chemistry. After sharing that I had earned a B, I was in shock to see a frown appear across his face. "Well that is not good enough, unfortunately," he stated.

Assured that he misheard me, I repeated myself, "Dr. Blackwood I said a B as in boy, not a D!" I laughed.

"I know what you said. Bs are not good enough and you shouldn't be content with this grade," he remarked.

"Well I know a lot of people who failed or got a C in this class, so I think a B is pretty good," I defended.

"Earning a B is an average grade. At Michigan, we are not looking for average physicians, we want outstanding physicians. Your goal should be to get an A. You should never be this excited about getting a B. Tamika, you're an A student who just got a B in Organic Chemistry and you're sitting there with a smile," he continued. "You're a closet 3.8 student. When are you going to finally come out the closet?"

"So students cannot get into medical school with a B on their transcript? I have heard otherwise. If that's how Michigan medical school is, then maybe I don't want to attend the medical school here." I was so offended by his lack of shared excitement with my good grades! I was extremely defensive in that moment. Because there were many people who I've heard of who failed Organic Chemistry the first time, or barely passed, or dropped the course and changed their major, I truly was proud that I got a B. In high school I would not have been as excited getting a B, but at the top public university in the country, I was damn proud of myself!

Dr. Blackwood replied, "Of course, students get into medical school with Bs on their transcripts. You need to stop comparing yourself to your peers in your classes. You keep forgetting that as a Black student, you have to work harder, get better grades, and excel more just to be looked at as equal. I'm not saying I am not proud of what you have accomplished. But I am saying that you cannot simply be content with this B. Would you be interested in taking the course over?"

"Taking the course over because I earned a B?" I paused. Maybe he was onto something. After all, he did sit on the admission committee for the medical school. I thought to myself, *let me breathe and think about what he is saying.* "Ok so if I took it over, I could definitely get an A. I almost got an A this time around. I don't really want to take it over, but if that's what it takes to get into medical school, I trust you and I am willing to do it." I wanted to be a doctor so bad that I would have done just about anything to secure my pathway.

He chuckled, "If you take the course over and get an A, that does not say much. It's your second time taking the course, so of course we expect you to ace it. If you want to impress admissions, take Organic Chemistry with honors and get an A. Then you may turn more heads. Just think about it."

I left his office that day and as soon as I hit the door to my apartment, I cried like a baby. Ugly cried. There I was, proud of my grades and how I had turned my GPA around from that C freshman year, had my parents pay for all these summer classes, and it still wasn't good enough. I was crushed to the core. I cried to my mom. Again to my dad. Cried to my roommate. I don't know how my tear ducts weren't sucked dry that semester because I cried more during that time than I ever had in my life.

Why was my best not good enough? How does he know this was not my best? How does he know that I am a "closet 3.8 student"?

Why do I have to work harder than my non-Black counterparts just to be considered "equal"? My parents had told me that growing up and I never understood why. Then I found myself in a situation where the concept was coming up again. *Maybe I should have kept down that business path. That advisor was right, I was not going to get into medical school at this rate...*

Nope.

The doorbell rang. I wasn't expecting anyone and Nita wasn't home. *Who would be coming to my apartment unannounced in the middle of the afternoon?* I looked in the peep hole. It was Shelley, one of my teammates from my dance team. She was a few years older than me and was working on her PhD. Shelley was one of the sweetest people I knew and didn't have a mean bone in her body. She was beautiful, driven, sweet, and one of the smartest people I knew. I hoped everything was ok. It was unlike her to pop up at my house in the middle of the day. I didn't want to answer the door because whenever I had been crying my face was beet red, with puffy eyes, and there was no hiding it. I figured it was something important so I opened up the door.

"Hey girl! What's up?" I tried to fake like I was in the best of moods. Shelley saw right through my theatrics.

"Oh my gosh, Tamika! What's wrong? Is everything ok? Do I need to come back?" she questioned with concern. She came into my apartment to drop off a shirt for our upcoming dance performance. I had completely forgotten about it and forgotten that I had given her my address and told her to come by that day, as I finished classes early that day. I wanted to thank her for the shirt, pay her, and have her be on her way, but for some reason, my tears came rushing out.

"I'm ok! I just had a really bad meeting with a mentor about my grades and he said that what I have been doing wasn't good enough for medical school. I feel like I have wasted my time here. This school is hard as hell and I have been busting my ass to maintain my grades and extracurriculars. I thought he would have been proud of me but instead he said that my grades weren't good enough," I started on my rant.

"Tamika, I know you are a believer, aren't you? Do you have faith in God?" she asked gently.

"Well of course I do, but..." I defended.

"But what? I know Michigan is hard. I am finishing up my dissertation and it's been quite the journey. When I first met you, you told me that you were pre-med and you had prayed about it and knew that was God's purpose for your life. Do you remember that?" she asked.

"Yeah, I do," I responded quietly.

"You have everything going for you. You have already encountered a lot to get here and to achieve what you have achieved so far. Why would God bring you to all of this if He didn't plan on bringing you through all of this? The road is bumpy and difficult but it certainly isn't impossible," she explained. Shelley was right. Those words stuck in my head the rest of my life. I had to think back on the level of confidence I had when I informed her that I wanted to be a doctor. It is easy to be confident and sure of yourself when everything is going well. The challenge was remaining positive and confident when everything was not going well. I had prayed about it so many times and received confirmation that I was on the path God had laid out for me. I needed to keep working hard and things would fall into place.

I think a common misconception with faith is that we feel if God has confirmed our calling or our purpose, we think it's going to be an easy path, with no resistance and continued open doors. That's just not true. He will see us through it according to His will, but it will take hard work, determination, and discipline on our behalf. I knew I had made a choice to become a doctor but it was a decision that I had to make every single day over and over again.

Shelley and I talked for just a short while and I instantly felt better and motivated. Her coming over that day was no coincidence and that conversation meant more to me than I am sure she ever even realized. I had many more situations when I needed to be "talked off a cliff," but by surrounding myself with great mentors filled with wisdom, optimism, and faith they have carried me through until I learned to be able to "talk myself off the cliff.

As soon as she left my apartment that day, I had to shake off those negative feelings immediately. *This is my dream and I am going to accomplish it.* Dr. Blackwood is an esteemed physician who knows exactly what it takes to get there. His blunt words and advice hit hard, but they were necessary.

Although my grades were *good*, I could not get comfortable with *just good* grades. I needed *exceptional* grades and that needed to be my goal every semester. His words have forever remained etched in my heart. Not just in my application to grades, but even as a physician. My goal is exceptional and when I arrive at exceptional, I need to go even further. Not only did I have personal goals to achieve, I had community goals to achieve too. We had barriers to break down and glass ceilings to break through. This little Black girl from Detroit wasn't going to be the anomaly who made it. I want it to be so common to see a woman physician, so common to see a Black physician, that when you introduce yourself as the doctor, it isn't a surprise. I want it to be so common to see Black female physicians that we no longer have a stereotype of what a doctor looks like.

By the time I began my senior year at Michigan, I had already taken the MCAT and was in the process of applying to medical schools. All of my pre-requisites had been taken except Biochemistry, which I was taking in the fall semester of senior year. This class was a beast and I was struggling to stay afloat. The first exam, I had bombed, and the second exam I had done really well. The third exam would be a grade determiner so I needed to do well again. I studied hard and met with the professor and put in all the work necessary to excel. The night before the exam, I received a call.

"Hey Tamika. Grandmother is still in the hospital and she is not doing well. You need to come home," my mom said in a very melancholic voice.

"Come home for what? I know she does not feel well but she is so strong, she always fights through. She will be fine. I will come home this weekend after I take my Biochem exam," I responded.

"Tamika, the doctors are very concerned about internal bleeding. They have instructed me to tell family to come in this time. It is not looking good," my mom paused. "If you have to take your exam first, that is fine, just come home after you take your exam."

Was this really happening? My grandmother was one of the closest people to me. She had a series of health problems that had led to chronic illness and frequent hospital admissions and "scares", but she always made it out ok. She was the strongest person I knew. The thought of her no longer being around made my entire soul numb. We have been told so many times by doctors on multiple occasions since I was in middle school that she was dying. There we were, 11 years later and she was still alive and kicking. The tone in my mom's voice was different this time. Even my heart felt different. I needed to go home and gave zero shits about my Biochemistry exam or class or even being a doctor at this point. I needed to see my Grammy. I sent my professor an email explaining why I wouldn't be taking the exam the next day, didn't wait for a response, hopped in my car and zipped back home.

My grandmother ended up pulling through and was eventually discharged home from the hospital. Thank you, Jesus. This one had me more shook than the other scares we had in the past and I was so relieved to see her bounce back again. When I say bounce back, I don't mean back to her baseline, but she was not in the hospital anymore. Her health was still in critical condition and continued to decline throughout my senior year of college. By the time I graduated from college, she was living at an in-patient hospice facility where I frequently visited her. She was so proud to know that I was finishing college and that I had been accepted into medical school.

"Guess what, Grammy? I am officially going to Meharry Medical College! I received my acceptance letter earlier today," I exclaimed while barging into her room.

"That is fantastic, baby! I never once doubted that you could do it," she shouted back.

"You know you are the reason I wanted to become a doctor. All the stories you told me about nursing school and your patients sounded so exciting. You had me interested since I was a little girl and that fire was never lost!"

My grandmother replied, "I am not the reason you chose to go to medical school. I am a nurse, not a doctor. I had no impact on you doing this."

I snapped back, "Are you joking?" My grandmother was notorious for joking around, using sarcasm, and being pretty blunt at all times. It's a legit question to ask if she was joking. "Most of my life has been spent talking to you about medicine—whether your nursing stories or with your doctors. I have watched you in the clinic, hospital, rehabilitation, and now hospice. I know your favorite doctors and your least favorite doctors and why. I know who has poor bedside manners and who doesn't. All the things you assumed I never paid attention to, I did. I want to encompass all the positive you see in them and make sure I am not anything like the negative. When I talk to families, I want to be honest yet compassionate and empathetic."

Since that was one of the last conversations I had with my grandmother, I do truly wonder sometimes if she was joking. *Did she know how much of an impact she had made on my career choice? Was she just being humble? Did I ever explained to her how much of an impact she had made on my decision to pursue a career in medicine?* She was my only exposure to healthcare growing up and she was one hundred percent my inspiration in becoming a physician. I just hope that she knew that before she passed away.

My grandmother died one week before I had to be in Nashville, Tennessee for my first day of medical school. I considered not going. My grandmother was the closest person to me. We were one and the same and she understood me to the core. I regretted being so caught up in trying to get into medical school in my last couple years of college that I did not see her as often as I used to. We talked on the phone frequently, but it decreased significantly when I was focused on school. My regrets turned into resentment. I resented my own dream of becoming a doctor. I was so enthralled in the process that I did not stop and spend time with my loved ones while still alive and that was a sting I could not shake. These are all the reasons why I did not want to go to medical school anymore, on top of the fact that my family needed me in Michigan. I was torn. I am the emotional and spiritual rock of my family and that time, they needed me. I could have stayed and gone to medical school in Michigan, as I had been accepted to a couple schools in state as well. That way I would be satisfying my dream and being there for my family. This was the best of both worlds. I wanted to be there for my family when they needed me, especially because as I had just learned about my grandmother's passing, and tomorrow is never promised.

I knew my grandmother would not want me to defer a year or not go to medical school altogether because of her passing, but it would be hard to move across the country alone, away from my family, grieving, and starting one of the most difficult curriculums in embarking on a medical degree. I prayed about it. I made the decision to go to Meharry Medical College in Nashville, Tennessee where I had told my grandmother I was going prior to her death. I packed whatever could fit in my black Ford Fusion and drove to Nashville for the first day of medical school. This was hands down the hardest decision I had made in my life and that day was full of emotion and tears in my family. My parents and I got into a big fight right before I left. Emotions were high and I didn't know if it was a result of that alone, or if my mother resented me for leaving her while she was grieving the death of her mother and best friend. My car was packed with lamps, clothes, and as much stuff as I could pack into the backseat and trunk and I made the decision to leave anyways, despite the intense argument we just had in our driveway. I had promised that I would be at the wake that would take place in a couple weeks in Florida and would get a plane ticket once I got settled. There's no way I was not going to attend my grandmother's memorial, as difficult as it was.

That moment was one of the heaviest moments in my life. I felt horrible leaving Michigan at a time like that with everyone grieving the loss of my grandmother. I was grieving as well. She was literally my second mom and I was hurting deeply on the inside but I expressed grief and pain very differently. I didn't talk about my feelings to anyone and from the outside, I probably looked like I was doing well. In actuality, I was drowning. I didn't have a therapist and wouldn't have been open to one at that age either. I felt the best way to deal with it was to not deal with it. I buried myself in everything else and tried not to think about it. It was probably the worst way to handle it and I didn't know better at the time. I was just trying to make it.

I entered into a depressive state that lasted pretty much my entire first year of medical school. So often had I dealt with mental health in an unhealthy way, that I had mastered "my cover up". To my friends, classmates, and family, I probably looked like I was doing just fine, but inside, I hated myself. I hated myself for not taking a year off, for leaving Michigan when my family needed me, and most importantly for not spending as much time with my Grammy in her last few years of life. I got so caught up in college life and trying to become a doctor that I had lost sight of the things and people who matter to me most. That was the toughest pill to swallow and every single day that I woke up and went to school, I resented my decision to become a doctor for that reason alone.

So often, we normalize dysfunction or unhealthy habits that we cannot recognize them when we are living and breathing them. My first year of medical school, I was so stressed out because of school and my depression I was secretly battling, it began to impact my body. I began having severe gastrointestinal issues which resulted in me vomiting, dry heaving, and feeling nauseous all the time. I didn't actually make an association with my stress until I finally went to see the doctor on campus. I thought it was pretty ridiculous to be in medical school, with access to every type of doctor at my fingertips, having medical problems, and not seek help.

After my consultation with an internist, they were concerned that my stress was causing the GI issues. He informed me that if I didn't get a better grip on my stress, it could worsen. He felt that I was having bad reflux and potentially a gastric ulcer. He wanted me to undergo an EGD, an electrogastroduodenoscopy. In short, he wanted to stick a camera down my throat to see what was going on. I adamantly refused it. I had never had any major procedures in my adult life and I didn't want to start! I asked if there were alternatives. He gave me a prescription for omeprazole, a medication to help with my reflux and ultimately said I needed to get a grip on my stressors. I had never been on prescription medication before so it was all pretty scary to me. Although the nausea and vomiting had worsened, it was something that I had "normalized" previously. I really had started experiencing these symptoms in college and inappropriately associated it with Wendy's chicken sandwiches. My roommate Nita used to be looking at me crazy when I would be doubled over vomiting or dry heaving randomly. I never sought medical advice—I just stopped eating Wendy's chicken sandwiches.

I took my doctor's advice and continued to work on stress relief, self-care, and exercising more. I worked out pretty regularly in college and since I had started medical school, I rarely went to a gym or did much physical exercise. Incorporating that back in during my first year helped a great deal and after a few months of consistency, my symptoms had gone away apart from having an occasional flare up. I remember in pathology when we saw pictures of a Barrett's esophagus and it resulting in esophageal cancer, I immediately cringed in my seat. *Was that what my esophagus looked like? Is that why my doctor wanted to do an EGD on me? Did he think my insides looked like that? Was I at risk for developing cancer?* I don't care what anyone says. Every first-year medical student becomes a hypochondriac transiently. You learn about so many different conditions and clinical symptoms and start to make diagnoses of yourself, friends, and family members. When your professor tells you the symptoms of a brain tumor, the next time you get a headache, you're convinced that you have a brain tumor and need imaging of the brain. When we were shown pictures of craniosynostosis, a condition when the sutures of your skull close prematurely forming an abnormal shape, you instantly start noticing the shape of your head as well as your classmates'. Every medical student goes through this phase which can be annoying to your close family and friends!

Once I got into a better routine and my GI symptoms subsided, I felt like I had "cured myself", but I still did not seek counseling. In hindsight, it would have been extremely helpful at that transition because I was still very much in a dark place and resenting "choosing my career" over my family. Just four years prior, I had regretted not standing up for my dream regardless of the situation. I felt the need to keep my promise to myself to never let anyone or anything stand in the way of me pursuing my dream. I dreamed of becoming a doctor, so I was going to do just that. I had a laundry list of reasons why I wanted to go to Meharry—including God sending me there—so I already knew what needed to happen. Even more importantly, that was where I told my grandmother I was going to attend before she passed away. I didn't even have housing in Nashville yet. I emptied out my savings account and stayed in a hotel for my first few weeks of medical school. Whatever it took to get my MD, I was going to do it. I can honestly say, looking back, that I am so glad that I made the decision to become a doctor and to attend Meharry Medical College. If I had made decisions based on my emotions, I would be sitting in a different pile of regret today.

Affirmation to recite: *I am going to defend my dreams at all costs. I will continue to put my all into achieving them.*

Question: *Can you remember a time when you took a leap of faith in the name of pursuing your dreams? What made you take that leap? Did you have any regrets afterwards?*

Part III

The Cocoon (Medical School)

CHAPTER 8

Umm... That's a Dead Body!

"You always have to remember to take care of yourself first and foremost because when you stop taking care of yourself, you get out of balance and you really forget how to take care of others."
—Jada Pinkett Smith

I parked in the on-campus parking garage as instructed in the welcome email. As I got out of my car and walked toward the stairwell, I ran into another young Black woman. She asked me, "Do you know where the orientation is at?"

I responded, "Um, not really, but I'm sure we can find it together."

Courtney who was there for her first day of dental school was the first person I met at Meharry Medical College. She has become a lifelong friend. We walked up the front steps of the LRC Building and hurried into our seats for orientation. I was in awe when I walked in the auditorium and looked around. It felt so good to see so many people that looked like me who were aspiring physicians, dentists, and researchers.

We had to introduce ourselves one by one around the room. I quickly learned the perks of going to a smaller school and being able to do things like this. Even still, there were almost 200 of us in the room, and it definitely took some time. Some students were shy, others made jokes, some were long winded, and others kept it short and sweet.

You may be thinking there is no way everyone would remember over 200 introductions, right? That's what I thought too, but to this day I remember a lot of people based on those introductions and where they were from, or what funny thing they said when it was their turn. You'd be surprised how much these things stuck with all of us. I remember one of my friends, Gray, told me a couple years later that he remembers the day I introduced myself. I said my name, where I was from, and my undergraduate college and my major. I majored in Brain, Behavior, and Cognitive Science at the University of Michigan. He explained how he was so impressed by my major and thought I was going to be stuck up and arrogant. Furthest from the truth. I laughed and explained, "It sounds fancy but it's basically just biopsychology." We shared a laugh.

That was the beginning of a journey we had no idea we were about to embark on together and I will cherish this day forever.

It may sound like all bells and whistles, but it was tough. That was my first time being in a foreign environment, no family nearby to call or visit. I went to class and studied then went back to my hotel I was staying in down the street.

I did not attend any of the "welcome" events everyone was attending. I pretty much kept to myself. This was unlike me, as I have always been a social butterfly. With the recent passing of my grandmother, feeling homesick, and scared about the journey I had signed up for, I was not exactly in the mood for meet and greets. One day during class, everyone was talking about going bowling that night. I loved bowling, but I wasn't interested in going with a bunch of strangers. I remember Brandon (the only person I knew in town) convincing me to come out and stop being anti-social. Brandon and I went to the same middle school, high school, college, and now we were in the same class in medical school. I felt comfortable enough that if he was going to be there, maybe I should come out of my shell. I'm the most extroverted introvert there is; never seemingly shy, always appearing outgoing and social. Deep inside, I don't like being out of my comfort zone for prolonged periods of time. I knew was going to spend the next four years with these folks, so I thought I might as well get to know them.

I went to the bowling alley and had a great time. A few of the friends I met that night, Lauren, Maya, and Kyzwana became lifelong friends that I still talk to today. On my way home, I got a flat tire. I instantly felt that void of having my family (i.e. my dad) nearby. My dad would have been so proud if I had remembered the basics he taught me of how to change a tire, but I didn't. I was in the hood with a flat tire and it was 1 AM. I called Brandon. Through our struggle, we met another classmate Kevin who stopped to help get the donut on my car. Moments like this that may sound insignificant, but it really warmed my heart. I expected Brandon to help as a long-time friend, but Kevin literally stopped and helped on the strength of us being all Meharrians and we are family and we are going to help one another. This was one of many moments at Meharry where I stopped in my tracks to be thankful for such a loving family to be a part of during such an arduous process.

Meharry was a four-year unexplainable journey. We worked hard, partied hard, and supported each other on the journey. It wasn't perfect. What family is? But I wouldn't trade the experience for anything. My affinity for the school ran so deep that I became a member of several organizations and committees. I wanted to help the school continue to stand as tall as it had been and I wanted the community to see how precious of a gem Meharry truly is.

Since I had attended the University of Michigan (a primarily White institution) for undergraduate, that was all I had to compare post-secondary education to and Meharry (a historically Black college) was very different for obvious reasons. Gross Anatomy is one of the first classes you take in medical and dental school. Cadavers are used to learn anatomical parts including muscles, nerves, blood vessels, lymph nodes, etc. At Michigan, I remember going into the lab a few times and looking at the prosections. A prosection is a body part that has already been dissected, fat taken out, veins, arteries, nerves, and muscles already cleaned out, and clearly identifiable with a label. I always had a good time going into the labs to learn about the body in depth at Michigan. This was the only anatomy experience I had to compare mine to.

Day one of Gross Anatomy Lab at Meharry, we broke into lab groups and were assigned to a table. I remember walking into the lab and seeing 30 to 40 dead bodies laying there, embalmed and cold. Nothing can mentally prepare you for that sight. *Wait, where are the prosections? These are full dead bodies with faces on them. Where are the tags and labels?* Dr. Jackson, our anatomy professor, explained to us that we do not use prosections at Meharry, but we will be dissecting the bodies in their entirety from skin to bone. We can use our Grey's Anatomy book or Netter's Atlas and find all the parts that are listed because they will all be on the exam. I was in disbelief. This is going to take forever! We only have a few hours of lab a day. "Well you better come in here after class, after dinner, in the middle of the night, whenever to get it done before the exams," he reported.

That was no exaggeration. Gross Anatomy was broken up into "blocks". Lower limbs, upper limbs, head and neck, etc. Blocks were about 4-6 weeks long and we had to not only study the material in the book, but identify the vessels, nerves, muscles, fascia in our body and then in other classmates' bodies as well during practical exams. I acquired a true appreciation for how "unique" we all are. This artery may be in one area on one body and a slightly different location on another body. So we had to not just memorize our body, but learn how the body parts coursed and the different variations. We also had to properly dissect the body, layer by layer and being careful not to cut something we have not identified yet. This taught me how to appreciate the scalpel and sharpened my innate surgical skills. I loved Gross Anatomy; the material, the lab, and most importantly, the instructor, Dr. Jackson.

He was so hard on me from day one, but he always believed in me from the moment he met me and watched me with my scalpel. He expected perfect scores on exams, especially the practical exams and he expected our body to be an example so he could show other students how to identify certain structures. He would intentionally tell us when another dissection at another table was further along or cleaner than ours, because he knew we, in true competitive fashion, would stay extra late that night to make sure ours was caught up. I'll never forget, after one of the exams, I went to Dr. Jackson's office to discuss my grade. I said "oh my gosh, I got a 93%! I thought I had failed that exam!"

His response with a poker face, "You should have earned a 100%!" Then he would smile and we would share a laugh. Despite the laugh, I knew he was dead serious. His expectations for me exceeded my own. He reminded me very much of Dr. Blackwood, my mentor from college. I was flattered by the high expectations, but it definitely gave me a few grey hairs. Literally.

I loved that my professors knew me by name. Not just me, but all of my classmates as well. They knew about our family, interests, our strengths and weaknesses. They stayed late for office hours, or came in at the crack of dawn to explain certain mechanisms to us. We even had some professors come in on the weekend to hold review sessions for the class. These are the things that I can never overlook about my experience at Meharry. I was used to being a number in a sea of students, rather than Tamika Cross, a young lady with potential to be an outstanding surgeon one day, as he frequently reminded me.

Dr. Jackson was a mentor to me and I am so blessed to have met him my first year at Meharry. He built up my self-confidence and kept me pushing through a process that was intimidating from day one. When he first met me, I wanted to be a pediatrician and he was upset because he said I was destined to be a surgeon. He was so proud and relieved when I told him 3 years later that I decided to go into OBGYN and would be putting my surgical skills to good use.

I could go on and on about the awesome experience I had at Meharry, but you get the point. Meharry helped me mature academically, personally, and even spiritually. I am so glad that I listened when God nudged me there because it was exactly where I belonged. Had I attended any other medical school, my experience would have been very different, and I may not have had the same outcome.

Ever since my first year of medical school, I wanted to do something surgical. I knew for Pediatrics, I would not be doing anything surgical unless I did some type of subspecialty. Subspecialty in Pediatrics meant the children would be pretty sick. From my shadowing in college in Pediatric Infectious Disease and hematology/oncology, I knew that my emotions likely could not handle that. I cried almost every time I left the hospital shadowing on these services.

"Tamika, what do you want to be when you grow up?" I was frequently asked this throughout all phases of my life. What student is not asked this? It's an important question to ask at a young age... to make kids dream, make them see that the sky is the limit and what interests and talents they have.

"I want to be a doctor or maybe a teacher" was my routine response. Sometimes it was doctor, sometimes it was teacher, and sometimes I just kept it real, that I really could see myself as either one. When I got older, the follow up question was added.

"What kind of doctor do you want to be?" they asked. My routine responses were either anesthesiologist or pediatrician. I did not know any anesthesiologists, so I honestly think I just liked the fact that I could say and spell the word. I barely knew what they did. But that was my response. I eventually dropped it because I knew nothing about the field except you put people to sleep and that sounded boring to me at that age. I became pretty consistent with my response that I wanted to be a pediatrician though. I absolutely loved children, babysitting, mentoring, tutoring... you name it. Almost all of my community service was geared toward children. I saw the power in youth my entire life and being a doctor just for the kiddos seemed to be up my alley for sure. I was matched with Dr. Blackwood, a specialist and pediatrician because I said I wanted to be a pediatrician. I went to medical school exclaiming that I wanted to be a pediatrician. I honestly thought I did. Until I was exposed to other fields.

Well if I did not do Pediatrics, what would I do? I told everyone, including my family, "I am not sure anymore what kind of doctor I want to be. But I know for a fact that I will never be an OBGYN!" My mom reminds me of this statement I made frequently in college and medical school, because she finds it hilarious that I am now a practicing OBGYN who is in love with her career. If I am being honest, I said that out of ignorance. I did not know much about the field except that they do PAP smears and deliver babies, and I hate going to my OBGYN. I loved her as a person but the process of getting completely naked, putting my legs spread eagle in stirrups, and having a doctor stick a speculum inside my vagina, look around, swab things, then insert her hand in my vagina, was not exactly a visit I looked forward to annually. *How could anyone want to do this to anyone? This is so invasive,* I thought. From my own experience and ignorance of all of what the field of OBGYN encompassed, I wanted to avoid liking that field at all costs. Then second year second semester happened.

Medical school is four years. The first two years are in the classroom, the last two are in the hospital on clinical rotations. By the end of your third year, you have to apply for residency in whatever field of medicine you chose, so you need to know what type of doctor you want to be. At the end of my second year of medical school, I was conflicted because I did not want to do Pediatrics anymore but I did not know what else I would do. I was leaning toward general surgery. I really wanted to be a surgeon since I enjoyed operating so much. The school matched us up to shadow on different clerkships at end of our second year to prepare us and expose us before our third year which would be our clinical years based in the hospital. A few of my friends and I decided to sign up for Labor and Delivery. I basically picked this out because I thought it would be cool to see a baby being born. None of us wanted to go into OBGYN, so we may never get to experience it outside of our OB rotation during third year. We wanted to stay together so Khaisha, Rich, Gray, and I signed up.

It was an amazing experience. We had a chance to see babies born, see patients in clinic, do ultrasounds on pregnant and non-pregnant women, watch surgeries of hysterectomies or removing fibroids from women or cysts on their ovaries. In the clinic, we got to talk to women about preventative health topics and educate our patients. Oh no. I LOVED THIS FIELD! I had no idea I loved OBGYN, but I certainly did. Everything about it was interesting and versatile. The fact that I could have continuity with my patients, perform surgeries, deliver babies, and see patients in clinic for routine check ups was mind-blowing to me. The doctor we were assigned to was Dr. Byrd. She was exactly the kind of doctor I wanted to be. Her patients loved her, she was very knowledgeable, and was well respected by the residents, students, and her colleagues. I found it amazing that in one day, an OBGYN could deliver a baby, tie someone's tubes, see patients in clinic, and perform an ultrasound and then do an emergent surgery for a large cyst. The versatility and adrenaline rushes made me fall in love. The crazy work hours, not so much, but when you love what you're doing, it's worth the struggle.

We worked in a community-based hospital with a large indigent patient population. We saw women from all walks of life. I remember sitting on the labor and delivery unit as a second year student and wondering what would make clinic visits a more enjoyable experience for women. The standard exam room was cold, with tile floors and paper gowns that stick to any nervous perspiration and tore at any quick movements. There were diagrams and posters on the wall about scary women's health topics. While women are waiting for their doctor to come in, they sat there, terrified, growing antsy by the second, and staring at random posters on the walls. While this experience is not much different from any other doctor's office, what was unique about the gynecologist office is that women knew that an invasive exam was about to take place. Women sat there completely naked, knowing in just a few moments, their gynecologist would be entering the room and requesting their feet to be placed in stirrups, with their legs spread eagle. I knew what women felt, because as a patient, I felt it too. I dreaded my annual exams. Regardless of how nice my doctor was to me, the experience was intimidating and uncomfortable.

Since we had long periods of downtime in between deliveries, I found myself daydreaming and meditating for long stretches at a time. I wanted to create a different experience one day. I thought it would be nice to create an OBGYN office that was warm, inviting, comfortable, and less intimidating. I wanted to create a clinic that had a full-service spa with massage therapy, facials, aromatherapy, etc. By creating a one-stop shop for women to relax and get their women's health exams taken care of would be amazing.

I wanted to create a spa that had services that were pregnancy friendly so my obstetric patients could indulge as well. I felt that this would be more encouraging for women to come in for their exams, and this unique experience would allow women to relax. As I sat there daydreaming about this experience, I added ideas to it over the course of the next 6-12 months. Because the idea seemed so far-fetched and unrealistic, I did not share my dreams with many people; only a couple close friends and my family.

Even if I could not build a joint OBGYN clinic and medspa, I knew there were a myriad of ways that I could make a difference in the life of my patients. Women are frequently the backbone of their families and spend countless amounts of hours and energy caring for everyone else. They are working full time jobs, coming home and cooking, cleaning, taking care of the kids, etc. Not to mention if a family member is ill, women are commonly the ones who are caring for those family members as well. Because women spend so much time putting everyone else before themselves, I saw women neglecting their own health. Even today, I find myself softly scolding my patients who have waited 10 years to get their mammogram, or PAP smear. Women who have had heavy bleeding during their periods and waiting years to go to the doctor for it—and usually that is after a major health event such as passing out. Many women are also embarrassed to go to the gynecologist because they do not want to talk about the foul odor in their vagina, or the cluster of bumps that popped up on their labia, or a married woman of 30 years requesting STD testing due to infidelity in the marriage. Teenage girls with infections and pregnancies do not come to the OBGYN because they are scared or embarrassed or ashamed if their parents found out. As a result, these infections worsen to the point that now she is hospitalized being treated for something that was an easy fix with a pill. Teenagers are going to dangerous heights to get abortions done by illegal back alley clinics because they do not want to tell their parents, or do not have the money or insurance to see a licensed physician.

These are only a few of the many areas of women's health that I knew I could make a difference in. Women deserve compassionate non-judgmental, non-government regulated, quality health care from health care providers who are relatable, approachable, and have their best interests at heart. Women deserve OBGYNs who are passionate about what they do and treat each patient like their own mother, daughter, aunt, sister, or grandma. Women's health is so important and I wanted to be an advocate for women and help close the gap between the health disparities that exist in this field. My passion and fire for this field was ignited in 2011 and that fire is still burning in me today.

***Affirmation to recite**: I have a purpose. My purpose is greater than me and once I find my purpose, I have the ability to change the world.*

***Question**: What is your purpose/calling? Do you feel that you are working in that purpose today? If you are, how many other people have you shared your journey with in efforts for them to discover their purpose? If not, what steps do you need to take to fulfill that purpose?*

CHAPTER 9

Failing Is Not an Option

"Success is to be measured not so much by the position that one has reached in life as by the obstacles which he has overcome while trying to succeed."

—Booker T. Washington

The traditional medical school curriculum is divided into two parts: basic science and clinical science. The first two years of medical school are your basic science years. This includes being in the classroom for more of a traditional educational experience with a series of lectures, labs, and exams. Typically, in the first year, a medical student will have Gross Anatomy and Physiology, Biochemistry, Pathology, Microbiology, Immunology, Genetics, and Pharmacology. For the most part, our schedule consisted of going to lecture everyday from 8 AM to 5 PM, study in the evenings, wake up and repeat again. Transitioning from college to medical school can be difficult because the course load is double on top of additional hours spent outside the classroom for clinical learning as well as studying. With so much material being jam-packed into the schedule, the pace is pretty quick as well.

Just like with any other academic program, every student has their strengths and their weaknesses. Microbiology was certainly my weakness. I remember sitting in the lectures confused as hell like, *how does this bacteria work? How does this virus work compared to this other virus?* I frequently found myself zoning out in lecture because it was not always making sense to me. I would go home and try to memorize the different bacteria and viruses and how they behave differently and ultimately be frustrated. Sometimes it clicked but most times, I sat there staring at my textbook for hours daydreaming and being frustrated with myself.

I had difficult classes before and I was able to buckle down, study, pass, and move on. This was different. I would study for hours and feel I had a better understanding, only to show up and bomb the exam. This course humbled me like none other. I had never struggled so much in a course. Now, I know you're probably thinking that I am the "gunner"; the student who is a perfectionist and overexaggerating about "failing" when I receive a B, as many medical students are perceived that way. As extra as I can be sometimes, let me give you some context to explain how serious I am about how I was struggling. I was failing! Yes, like studying my ass off, grinding, attending every class, feeling decent about my knowledge and receiving an F on my first exam. As much as I would have wished, no exaggeration here.

How was I going to become a doctor without passing Microbiology? Well, I wasn't. This is a required course in medical school and there was no way I would be able to advance to my second year of medical school without passing this class. I questioned the hell out of myself. *Was I fit to be a doctor? Was this a sign from God that I chose the wrong career path? Was I going to be thrown out of medical school? Do they have summer school in medical school? Would I have to repeat the whole first year if I failed microbiology?*

It's normal to have all of these feelings, and to be quite honest, most medical students have thought of quitting at some point in the journey. I knew that everyone who started medical school did not finish, but I didn't think that was ever going to be me. Many people never do. I was doing well in my other courses so I didn't know how this would be handled if I failed the course. We had three exams, and a subject board at the end of the course. When there aren't many factors going into your grade, each component is worth so much. I improved on my second exam, but was still struggling and did not receive a passing grade. It came down to me having a one on one with my professor, Dr. Lima. I met with her during her office hours one day at lunch.

"Tamika, at this point in the course, we have to let students who are failing know where they stand and the potential consequences. You come to class daily, ask and answer questions, come to office hours, but your exam scores are really low. Is everything ok?" she questioned. *What did she mean by that? Did she think I was ill or had family problems going on? Were my grades that bad that she knew there was some extenuating circumstance that was bringing my grades down and causing me to perform poorly?* As much as I would have enjoyed blaming it on something personal, the truth was I just didn't have a thorough understanding of the material. With memorization and using test taking strategies, I was able to get some questions correct, but it truly didn't "click". I explained that to her and that everything was ok, I was just failing. Disappointed, she told me that I needed to do better.

"Well, Tamika, I hate to have to tell you this, but if you fail this course, we are offering it again in the summer. How are you doing in your other classes?" Dr. Lima asked.

"I'm passing my other classes. I didn't realize there was summer school here." I responded softly.

"If you're passing your other classes, you would just have to take my class over this summer. It isn't too big of a deal, but you definitely have to pass it before being allowed into your second year classes," She said. "As we are nearing the end of the course, there is only one final exam left and a subject board exam. You must ace the final exam and do exceptionally well on the board exam to be able to pass this course."

Ashamed, I lowered my head. I was embarrassed. It's not that I felt invincible like I could never fail a course, but I had never failed a class in my life before. I had worked my ass off to get to medical school, and there I was in my first year and already having a talk about receiving an F and having to attend summer school. I wondered if other students in my class were having the same difficulty. In medical school, you have a bunch of arrogant nerds who never want others to see them sweat. The biggest flex in medical school was acting like an exam was easy or like you had done exceptionally well. Classmates would walk out the exam smiling from ear to ear and turn to one another saying, "Well that wasn't too bad, was it?"

I later realized that this was more of a gauge to see how other students did or felt, and not a true representation of how said student performed. I never understood the need to lie and flex about grades. My policy was I don't discuss them. Whether I had aced an exam, or failed it, I didn't discuss my grades and I definitely didn't discuss how I "think" I did immediately after, prior to the grades being posted. I learned in medical school that you could feel great about an exam and confident about your grade, only to find out that you didn't perform as well as you thought you did.

I wasn't there to compare myself to others anyways. I just wanted to run my best race and finish strong. When classes are graded on a bell curve, many find that asking others helped them gauge how well they did. If everyone struggled with the exam, then the curve would be set lower, but if everyone did well, then it would be higher. So in essence, I understand the competitive spirit in bell curves. What I didn't understand was how asking another student how they felt after the exam was going to change your grade.

All exams had already been submitted, and whatever you earned, you earned already. Plus, with so many of them lying about their performance, it was just best to wait for the grade to be posted. Despite not discussing these things with classmates, I still wondered how other students fared. In that moment of extreme struggle, I wanted to be comforted in knowing that I wasn't just dumb, and that the course was difficult for others too. But it essentially did not matter, because whether there were three other failing students or 20, it would not change me having to retake the course in the summer.

I knew it was unlikely to be failing everything up until that point then pull off an A on the final and board exam, but I had to convince myself it was possible in order to keep pushing. Even once I got over the fact that I may earn my first F on my transcript, I was more upset because I had summer plans! With medical school being such a rigorous curriculum, you don't have traditional holiday and summer breaks. You may get some time off here and there, but as for summer, I knew that my only "summer off" was the upcoming one between first and second year. There is some time off from class between second and third year, but usually, that limited time is spent studying for the United States Medical Licensing Exam (USMLE) Step 1.

There are three steps in the medical licensing process: Step 1 is taken between second and third year of medical school, Step 2 is taken between third year and fourth year of medical school, and Step 3 is taken during your first year or two of residency. Passing Step 1 and 2 is required prior to graduating medical school and the scores are factored in when applying for residency programs early in the fall of fourth year. With that being said, since there was a true gap in classes between first and second year, many students used that time to vacation with friends and family and rejuvenate, or perform research. Research wasn't a requirement in my medical school, but it was highly encouraged. When applying for residency programs, research on your resume is favored, and it being relevant to the field in which you are applying is an added bonus.

I wanted research experience for a resume builder, but I also wanted the experience. I was interested in clinical research so I knew that I would likely engage in clinical research later on in my career as a physician. I wanted to do basic science research, in a lab, with mice. Watching science shows and movies growing up, when I thought of research, I had always thought of bench work; in a laboratory mixing chemicals, testing out different treatments, etc. I knew that ultimately I didn't have a long-term interest in it, but I'll try anything once and I wanted that experience for personal and professional reasons.

Because so many medical students across the country were also thinking similarly as far as gaining research under their belt for resume building, those research positions were hard to come by. We had to find a lab to work in that had openings available, and preferably so your summer isn't miserable, in a field that you are interested in or passionate about. You could also get a stipend for performing the research so that was an added bonus to a broke medical student who is knee deep in debt and could use a nice check to get by until the next refund check deposited in your account in the fall. I had landed a great position in a lab back home, at my alma mater, the University of Michigan.

Although I wasn't sure of what field of medicine I wanted to practice in at the end of my first year, my passion for helping minorities and children was very clear. For that reason, I chose to work in a lab under a pediatric hematologist oncologist doing sickle cell anemia research. Sickle cell anemia is a disease that primarily affects minorities, and although a lot of research had been performed in the field, there were many marks to be made in this department and I wanted to be a part of it.

In joining someone's lab, you hop onto their project and test out their hypothesis. I helped with running tests and labs on mice with sickle cell anemia. Our goal was to find a better treatment for sickle cell patients. Sickle cell anemia is a hemoglobin disease that results in flawed red blood cells with inadequate oxygen carrying capacity. As a result, instead of taking the shape of a normal red blood cell like a circular disc, sickle cell patients get red blood cells that turn into a sickle-shaped cell looking similar to a crescent moon. As a result of this new shape of the red blood cells, they can get stuck in the blood vessels, resulting in decreased blood supply and oxygenation of tissues, infarction, and necrosis or dying of the tissue. This process is extremely painful resulting in pain crisis that typically lands sickle cell patients in the hospital. If you've ever witnessed a patient having a sickle cell crisis, it is absolutely horrible. The amount of pain they are in is indescribable.

Due to sickle cell disproportionately affecting minority patients, with 90% of sickle cell patients being of African descent, this results in minorities in the emergency room frequently with pain crisis. Due to the systemic racism and bias, these patients are often met with skepticism, neglect, and misdiagnosis as "drug-seeking patients."

In the medical world, patients who come to the hospital with exaggerated or feigned symptoms in order to receive narcotics are labeled "drug-seeking patients". It is important to understand when you have a patient that is drug seeking because they are trying to get a "fix" or a "high" for their addiction, but don't actually require the $30,000 work up that many of us would like to do in trying to identify their underlying cause. Sickle cell patients are frequently thrown into that category as drug-seeking patients because many doctors or nurses do not believe the patients are in that much pain. It becomes a major issue when patients are getting different treatment depending on their ethnicity. There are studies that have proven this notion.

In fact, a study[1] in the American Journal of Emergency Medicine reported that Black patients are 40% less likely to receive pain meds than White patients and Hispanic patients were 25% less likely to get pain meds than White

---

1 Lee P., Le Saux M., Siegel R., et al. Racial and ethnic disparities in the management of acute pain in US emergency departments: meta-analysis and systematic review. *Am J Emerg Med* 2019; 37(9):1770–7. (http://bit.ly/2Lyqk3Q American Journal of Emergency Medicine, online June 5, 2019)

patients. In a 2016 study[2] published in the Proceedings of the National Academy of Sciences of the United States of America, 40% of first and second-year White medical students reported the belief that "Black people's skin is thicker than White people's." This is representative of the physicians employed at the hospitals (now) denying sickle cell patients in the middle of a vaso-occlusive crisis of any pain medications due to the inherent belief that they are addicts or are exaggerating their pain.

I wanted to join a team that was going to help find a cure or at least a treatment to help the disease to be more manageable in the interim. Since I had landed a spot working on this amazing project at my alma mater, I then had the opportunity to go back home for the summer with family and friends, stay rent free with my parents, and save the stipend I receive for the research. It made me extremely excited for the upcoming summer. If I failed Microbiology and had to repeat it in summer school, not only would I have to forfeit my research position, stay in Nashville alone, and not get my stipend, but I would have also had to break the news to my mentor, Dr. Blackwood, who helped me secure this research position. He and I had come a long way, and I remember the days I used to cry leaving his office all too well. There was no way that after he was so proud of me getting into medical school, that I could come back and

---

2 Hoffman K.M., Trawalter S., Axt J.R., Oliver M.N. Racial bias in pain assessment and treatment recommendations, and false beliefs about biological differences between blacks and whites. *Proc Natl Acad Sci U S A* 2016; 113:4296–301

tell him that I failed a class and was in summer school. He also put his neck out there in vouching for me as a highly intelligent, hardworking student who would be an asset to work in the sickle cell lab. *What was I going to do?*

I wasn't ready to throw in the towel yet. Although I wanted to, I knew I needed to fight until the final day of class. I couldn't keep doing what I had been doing though. I studied, read, attended class, went to office hours occasionally, and was failing. Insanity is doing the same thing over and expecting a different result. I had to get creative. I remember crying to my mom about my situation and we searched for alternative plans. She knew nothing about the medical field or medical school but my mom is one of the most resourceful people I know. We got online and searched for different microbiology books that helped break things down in a different way. We read hundreds of reviews and bought the books. These weren't the required textbooks for the class, but the required textbooks weren't teaching me shit so I had to get creative.

I spent several hours making flashcards, color coded charts, and spent every ounce of free time in between classes reviewing the material over and over. The new book I had truly simplified Microbiology in a different way and helped me classify the bacteria and viruses into groups or families to better understand them. Why hadn't I done this before? I also met with Dr. Lima every few days for the remainder of the semester to review what I had learned and she would quiz me in her office to make sure I understood.

I appreciated that about her and many of my professors at Meharry. They were truly invested in our careers and would bend over backwards to meet with us whenever we needed to ensure our success.

I had made it clear to Dr. Lima that I couldn't get an F and I needed to perform my summer research. As a researcher herself, she had so much respect for the field, and understood my drive. She never once doubted that I could get an A, even though I was very doubtful. A failing student doesn't go all semester failing then pull an A at the end; that just didn't make sense, especially because my hard work was resulting in an F! What I failed to realize was that because I took a completely different approach and was using different textbooks and learning methods and online videos, much to my surprise, I pulled off that A! I was able to pass the course and attend my summer research job back in Michigan.

That was when I realized that sometimes the "cookie cutter" approach doesn't work for you. The curriculum was structured in a way that helped many students to be successful in learning and understanding microbiology, but I was the minority and it didn't work for me. I had to create a strategy that worked for me. Everyone learns differently and sometimes a unique approach is needed to reach success.

Summer had arrived and I was back home in Detroit. Since my research job was in Ann Arbor, about 45 minutes from my parents' house, I had to get up early to commute back and forth in rush hour traffic, but it was worth it. After a long crazy first year of medical school, I wanted nothing more than to be around childhood friends and my family. There was no exam for me to study for and no assignments for me to catch up on and I could truly enjoy my job as well as my free time to hang with friends. I desperately needed that break.

While I wasn't exactly sure how well I was going to like bench research, it was an experience that I wanted under my belt. When I had talked to my principal investigator (PI), Dr. Baldwin prior to me starting, he had informed me that we would be working with mice. I was excited and terrified at the same time. I didn't know how my commute was going to be from my parents' house, so on my first day, I left a two-hour window just in case. As I exited the freeway at Main Street, a feeling of nostalgia filled my heart. Just a year ago, I was a pre-med student finishing up my bachelor of science degree, and then I found myself returning to my alma mater as a rising second-year medical student.

I was meeting him in the front lobby of the medical school, and I knew exactly how to get there. Being in the Black Pre-Medical Association in college, all of our meetings were held in the University of Michigan medical school. I think the reasoning behind that was twofold: convenience for our medical student and resident mentors, but also for us to experience the medical school lecture hall. Many of us do not always realize the impact of our environment. Sitting in the same seats as medical students and residents when I was a college student was extremely empowering. It made my dream feel it was within arm's reach. It also helped us become familiar with the layout of the medical school and the resources it had to offer. Walking those halls even though it was after hours, made me feel like I was a medical student. Although I wasn't, I knew that one day I would become a medical student, then resident physician and so on.

I headed to my usual place to find parking when I went to the medical campus at Michigan—the neighborhood. Parking on campus was extremely tough and expensive. The best parking was finding a spot in the surrounding neighborhoods, although you knew you would have to endure a lengthy walk to wherever you were going. I wasn't the only one with that novel idea, it was a well-known fact to all 40,000 students on campus, so finding a parking spot, even far, was still difficult. I found a spot finally and it was about a half mile away from the medical school. Not too shabby for Michigan's campus! Now you see why I always factored in a lengthy commute time between driving and walking a nice distance from wherever I landed a parking spot that day. This was a daily ritual Monday through Friday, but it was summertime, and the weather was beautiful, as was the campus, so I enjoyed the walks as they were therapeutic and time for me to meditate. I walked to the front doors of the medical school, took a deep breath, and entered. I felt proud. Even though this wasn't my medical school, and I had been denied admissions to Michigan's medical school, I was proud to be a medical student and invited there to perform research with one of the top researchers in the country.

I stood around while I waited for Dr. Baldwin. I had never met him in person, but I had looked up his picture, and he was a Black man with a bald head. That description would jump out to me with the limited diversity in the medical school. As soon as it turned 8 AM, I looked up and saw a bald Black man turn the corner. He looked exactly like his picture!

"Hi! I'm Tamika Cross, your medical student who will be working in your lab this summer! Very nice to meet you!" I introduced myself, reaching out to shake his hand.

"Nice to meet you finally, Tamika! I am happy to have you join our team! Let's head to the lab so I can show you around. I have another student working with me this summer, but she is out of town this week, so it'll be just you and me!" he said. Great! This would afford me time to pick his brain about the project and have one-on-one time to learn more about the research. After we reached the end of a few long hallways, we made a left into the lab. The lab looked just like the ones I had been in while taking my science labs as prerequisites to get into medical school. Black countertops, high office chairs on wheels, stools, and tons of expensive equipment. There was another researcher on the other side of the lab, but he wasn't there at the time. We headed over to his area in the lab.

"This is pretty cool! How often do you come here? I know you mentioned that you still see patients in the hospital and clinic, so how do you have time to come here too?" I asked.

"Different days of the week I work in the clinic, and others I am here working on my research. I typically always have patients in the hospital so I usually round on them in the morning or during my lunch break. This summer, we will get you to join me a few times so you can see what I do outside of the lab. Our main focus will be to get you some experience working in the lab though. Are you interested in becoming a pediatrician?"

Dr. Baldwin was extremely personable, approachable, and could carry an interesting conversation. The stereotypes of scientists were that they were weird, anti-social, and didn't interact with people much, as they were always in their lab. Dr. Baldwin was different. He had a family, went on vacation, saw real patients in the hospital and clinic, and overall seemed like a well-rounded guy.

"I always wanted to be a pediatrician because I love children. However, I am now entertaining the idea of other specialties. General Pediatrics seemed boring to me, and all the specialties in Pediatrics meant that the kids would be super sick, and I don't know if my heart could take that." I was honest. "How do you work with children and see them in so much pain and suffering every day? With you being a hematologist and an oncologist, I know you see quite a bit of cancer patients who are young. I don't think I could do it."

"You know, Tamika, a lot of people say that, but it's more rewarding than you think. I don't just have sad stories, I have the best victories too when my patients beat their disease. My career has shifted to working more with sickle cell patients than the full breadth of heme/onc. Seeing kids fighting this painful disease is my why. It makes my research so much more meaningful when I see the many kids I will be able to help if I can find a way to help their cells not to sickle," he replied.

He had a great point. Since he saw the clinical side as well as the bench research, it was full circle for him. If I had patients that I know my research could help, it would be that much more rewarding every day I step foot into the lab. It serves as a constant reminder of why it is so needed.

He had emailed me a few papers from other researchers to read prior to my first day so it would give me some background as to what sickle cell anemia is, how it works, and the targets for research. The next day, he spent half the morning explaining to me what his research was on. Patients with sickle cell anemia have red blood cells that take on a sickled or crescent moon shape rather than a pliable round disk. As infants, we have fetal hemoglobin which is comprised of four subunits; two alpha units and two gamma units. In adult hemoglobin, it is comprised of four units as well, but with two alpha units and two beta units. Over time, our fetal hemoglobin decreases and adult hemoglobin rises until you have primarily adult hemoglobin. With sickle cell patients, the abnormality targets the beta subunits which is seen in adult hemoglobin. Since sickle cell doesn't affect fetal hemoglobin, most patients with sickle cell have a protective automatic response where their body maintains fetal hemoglobin longer than a non-sickle cell patient. His research was targeting a specific transgene that would induce more fetal hemoglobin in sickle cell patients. With an elevated amount of fetal hemoglobin, the patient would result in less sickled cells, and an improved disease course. There was a treatment on the market that does that, but this was using a different method to target the gene that turns on for more production of fetal hemoglobin even in older patients. I thought this was the coolest thing on earth and couldn't wait to contribute to what sounded like a very promising project.

He had tons of mice, a third of which had sickle cell anemia, a third that had sickle cell trait, and a third that did not have either. Sickle cell trait patients meant they were carriers of the disease but did not actually have it. This results in more mild symptoms typically but sickle cell disease could be passed on to their children if they had children with a spouse that also carried the trait. He had other teams that worked on the mice as well and would put the transgene in the mice to see what happens. Typically, sickle cell mice had enlarged livers and enlarged spleens until eventually the spleen would then become small and nonexistent as a result of the disease's effects. So when it was time for us to assess the mice, we had to euthanize them, cut them open, take out their organs, weigh them, as well as collect their blood to run tests on them. We also took the data and entered it into an Excel spreadsheet. The other student and I assisted with this.

I remember when he asked me to pass him one of the mice, and my heart sank. *Pass you a mouse? Like pick it up and hand it to you? How do you pick up a mouse?* At the point he had requested this favor, I had been working with him for about a week and had seen him grab several mice. He just picked them up by the tail, but he wore thick gloves because some of them would bite when you have to reach into a large tank filled with squirming mice.

"Tamika, it's simple, just grab the tail and pass me that mouse right there," he demanded. I was terrified but I didn't want to show it. He couldn't know that I was scared of these squirmy animals. "Just make sure you grab them tight, some of them can get away fast." *Lord, the more he said, the more antsy I became.* He sensed my hesitation. He took a deep sigh as if he was annoyed and was about to grab the mouse himself, when I reached into the bin and grabbed the mouse and sat it down on his work area.

"Thanks! Not too bad was it?" he laughed.

"Not at all!" I lied. I was going to have to get over this if he was going to be expecting me to touch these mice. I knew previously that this project involved me working with mice, but I had never wrapped my head around the fact that I was going to have to touch the damn things! I hated "mice days", and preferred to just run the tests on the organs and blood back in the lab and do the data entry, but I wanted a good evaluation and possibly a letter of recommendation later, so I had to suck it up.

One thing I learned as a student was to secure a possible letter of recommendation from every experience you participate in. You never want to close lines of communication because you may need them one day. If you volunteer at a health clinic, or health fair, shadow a doctor, work in a lab, etc., always secure a "letter writer". I always encourage my mentees to do this very thing with every experience. I will advise that if you want a robust letter of recommendation, you need your letter writer to know you. Volunteering for a one-day health fair and asking for a letter of recommendation may not produce the strongest letter. After all, they just met you that morning. The best letters come from people who worked alongside you intimately for a long enough period of time to know your work ethic, character, personality, etc., because those are things that need to be included in a strong letter of recommendation.

Of course if you don't have those experiences, get what you can, but if you know up front, it is important to create those experiences where you can secure a strong letter of recommendation whether it be to aid in getting into college, medical school, or residency. This is also applicable to other fields outside of medicine. Admissions committees can tell if the person who wrote the letter just met you or has known you for several months or years; so always try to get a strong letter from someone who genuinely knows you.

The rest of the summer in the lab went really well. Dr. Baldwin kept his promise and allowed me to shadow him a few times in the clinic and hospital to visit his patients with him. Even with me not knowing the patients, it made our research feel meaningful. These adorable children were born with such a devastating and painful disease. Most of them were extremely mature for their age and knew more about their disease than I did as a medical student. They didn't complain about the disease or report how "unfair" it was for them to be born with it. I cannot imagine battling a chronic illness as a child and spending half of your childhood in and out of the hospital and doctor's offices.

I was honored to have secured this position with a great mentor and hardworking team. That summer, we made history in that our hypothesis was supported and we were able to induce the sickle cell mice's fetal hemoglobin, which was our goal! Although the research was nowhere near my idea, or my project, working on the project for those eight weeks where major advances were made in sickle cell anemia research was such a proud feeling. Dr. Baldwin was so excited that major barriers had been broken down with his research. He explained to me that he would be publishing the research later that year!

I spent more time doing graphs and charts to show the impressive differences we had made with the project. I had to present my summer research project when I went back to Meharry, so I needed clean charts and graphs for my board as well. When I think back on how my motivation to participate was mainly to gain research experience, I ended up loving it, and was able to be a part of a solid research team who made significant progress that summer.

Sometimes the goals we achieve are not necessarily the goals we set out to achieve. In this case, my experience proved to be way more exciting than I had expected. I didn't realize how much I was going to enjoy the lab, running the tests, or even working with the mice when I got over my fear. In order to achieve growth, we must sometime be forced outside of our comfort zone. If I had never taken a chance and tried an experience that I didn't think I was going to like very much, I would have never discovered my love and passion for research. Had I failed Microbiology, I would have landed myself a spot in summer school and missed out on this opportunity of a lifetime. I knew that failing wasn't an option; not because I knew the research experience was going to be as amazing as it turned out to be, but once I made up my mind to do something, I very seldom backed out. It was important to me as a woman of integrity to keep my word to assist in his lab. He had turned down other applicants to choose me, and he was getting free labor that summer as he didn't have to use his grant money to support me, because my school did.

That summer I learned the importance of keeping an open mind, even if you think your mind is already made up. With my scare of almost failing a class in my first year of medical school, I learned that everyone's experience and learning style is different. If the cookie cutter approach is not working for you, find another way to learn before it is too late. Don't be too proud to seek extra help, buy extra textbooks, or create a completely different studying technique compared to what your classmates have. Whatever works for you is the best approach, and no one can teach you that. You must learn that yourself.

> ***Affirmation to recite:*** *Nothing is impossible or too difficult for me. If I want it badly enough and my actions support that, I will achieve my goal!*

> **Question:** *Was there ever a time that a goal seemed so farfetched, that you almost gave up hope, but somehow continued down the path and you actually achieved it?*

CHAPTER 10

Doctors are Broke

"When you want something, you have to be willing to pay your dues."

-Les Brown

Doctors are in the top 1% of earners in the United States, making on average, about $196,000 each year. Now this figure varies depending on specialty, location, years of experience, etc., but this is the overall average. That's a pretty decent salary, huh? So why on earth is this a recurring hot topic? Why are doctors saying that they are underpaid when they make more money than 99% of Americans? Are these thoughts that have crossed your mind before? If not, it's probably because you're a physician as well! Ha!

Let's dive in. As a physician, one can work in a private practice, which can be independently owned or hospital owned, or work for a health care system. The job duties and salaries are very different among those two categories alone. Doctors who work for a health care system usually work for a large academic center or medical school, or for a hospital system. These doctors are usually salaried and make the same amount of money if they see five patients a day or 50 patients a day. The pay structure can sometimes include productivity bonuses that pay physicians that exceed certain thresholds.

I'm going to oversimplify it and say it's structured so that if you work more, you get paid more. This pay structure is more favorable to the physician that is a powerhouse and getting in several patients a day either in clinic or surgery. This is not so favorable for the physician who may be just as good of a doctor but sees less patients in a day, but is spending more time with each one. Doctors in private practice get paid based on productivity. See more patients and generate more money, they take home more money. Again, an oversimplification, but for our purposes, let's rock with it.

For several decades, insurance reimbursement has been on a steady decline. What that means is that the money doctors get paid for delivering a baby is significantly lower today than it was several decades ago. Typically, when it comes to prices, things increase with inflation, but insurance companies are managing to get away with paying less and less for the exact same services and sometimes they manage to not pay at all. I may be a bit biased, but can you imagine working for two weeks, then you receive your paycheck and its $0. You go to your boss who said that he or she decided they weren't going to pay you for the services you had already performed? Well just like you, physicians have bills, rent, mortgages, and car notes to pay, so for starters, that's a huge slap in the face!

With the reimbursement for each patient being significantly lower as time progresses, doctors are needing to squeeze more patients onto his or her schedule to be able to pay the overhead for the office. Doctors who work for large systems or institutions are pressured to schedule more patients per day in hopes that there will be enough revenue coming in to pay the staff, the light bill, the phone bill, purchasing supplies, etc. So when patients complain that they are waiting long periods of time to see their doctor, the truth is that the doctor is probably double or triple booked or behind on patients.

If a doctor has 10-minute appointment slots per patient, this includes the time they are checking your weight, blood pressure, and performing your exam. So how much time does that leave for you to address your multiple concerns you've waited six weeks to talk to this doctor about? Two minutes? Three minutes? How unrealistic is that? Patients deserve to have more time with their doctors.

The truth is that most doctors want to spend more time with each patient, but fear that too much time spent with one patient will lead to them having to shut their entire practice down. I know I may sound like I'm exaggerating. I wish that I was. Private practices are shutting down all over this country due to decreased reimbursements, and doctors cannot fit in enough patients to keep the lights on and pay their staff. Crazy, right? Some doctors who manage to fit all the patients in are zooming through the appointments with two to three minutes to talk. Sometimes for a routine check up, that may be adequate, but in most cases, patients want to feel heard, and no one likes a doctor running in, doing a speedy exam, and running out. I'm not giving doctors excuses for poor bedside manners and rushed clinic visits, but I am explaining the root of a much bigger issue.

Have you ever wondered why your doctor's surgery schedule is filled so far out? With the decline in reimbursements from insurance companies, surgeons are being paid even less for surgeries, regardless of when they are time consuming and complex. The math breakdown for this, is that in the time they are doing a 2 hour surgery, they could have seen at least 5 patients and generated more money than they would have received for the surgery. Due to this unfortunate fact, many surgeons only have so many slots per day/week as they know their productivity in clinic will be rewarded more money.

With less money being paid to doctors who go through, on average, 12–13 years of post-secondary education, along with the many stressors and costs associated with it, the field of medicine is becoming less favorable to people. The truth is, we have a shortage of doctors in this country, specifically in primary care. How the hell are we going to recruit more doctors by giving them less pay for more work, after spending the first 30 years of their life in school, along with empty bank accounts, and six figures in debt? Does that sound favorable to you? My guess is no.

Because of this very reason, I tell my mentees very bluntly that if they are going to be a doctor for the money, don't bother. You can make much more money, quicker, without six figures in debt in other industries. What keeps most of us going is either our passion or insanity.

Society has this unrealistic perception of doctors being wealthy, when the majority of us are not. Despite our six-figure salaries, wealth is defined by the difference between assets and debt. With six figures worth of debt, and minimal assets acquired, most doctors are living paycheck to paycheck. Regardless of the optics, we are not in a much better financial situation than the 99% of Americans that we make more than. Please don't be fooled by the media, I'm speaking facts and from experience.

Over the past five decades, doctors have earned about the same amount of money when taking inflation into consideration. However, despite the stagnant salaries of doctors, the cost of medical school tuition has sky rocketed. So if we are paying more money for school, taking out higher loans, but not being paid any more money for it, then guess what happens? Doctors are spending a lifetime trying to pay back their student loans and are coasting through life with a negative or very low net worth. By definition, that's not wealthy at all. It is much more widely accepted that "teachers are underpaid" than "doctors are underpaid". While I believe both to be true as both are inherently important jobs, most Americans do not believe the latter. Most Americans do not think that doctors are underpaid. Would you believe me if I told you that doctors earn three dollars an hour less than teachers when looking at lifetime earnings? If you need to see this for yourself, look at my diagram 1, 1.1, and 1.2 in the appendix.

Now that you have looked at my diagram, I want to drive home one more point. What does this financial picture look like for minority physicians? When it comes to many things along this journey, we finish last. Gender and racial pay gaps exist in almost every industry, so I know it should not be surprising when I say that a White male doctor makes more money than a Black female doctor. Without even diving into the etiology behind this fact, let's look at how this impacts the financial pictures mentioned above. As we close the gender gap representation in medicine, one may say it's surprising to know that women are still being paid significantly less money. If you're Black and a female physician, the outlook is dismal, as we are always in last place.

While I've expressed that medical student debt is substantial across the board, there is a disproportionate amount of debt experienced by Black medical students. So what happens when Black students are incurring more debt only to become a doctor that is getting paid significantly less than their White counterparts? Black medical student enrollment declines. Less Black students are willing to take that dive into a tense financial situation knowing that there is a strong possibility that paying that debt off could take the majority of their life. This is exactly what happened. Black medical student enrollment has declined, and as a result, our chances of closing the racial gap among doctors is becoming more and more unrealistic. Studies have shown that Black patients are more compliant when they have a Black doctor and that outcomes of Black patients is significantly better than when they are cared for by non-Black doctors. Despite the fact we have been living this public health crisis for decades, we are finally beginning to see more being done about it. In the fall of 2020, when racial health disparities were again making headlines with the COVID-19 pandemic, many large donations were made to Historically Black Colleges and/or Universities that train 80 percent of this country's Black doctors. This is a step in the right direction for Black students who are aspiring physicians. As for us who already fought the fight and endured the debt, we are just going to have to suck it up and hope for an increase in generational wealth for our children and grandchildren.

I am not discouraging Black students from becoming Black doctors. We actually need more Black doctors to be able to effectively treat our patients in our communities. I'm not discouraging any student from becoming a doctor. We need you! I'm simply saying that your reason has to be beyond the dollar signs. Become a doctor because of your passion. If you're doing it for the money, you are in for a rude awakening.

Affirmation to recite: *Passion fuels purpose. Passion fuels success. I am passionate about ___________.*

Question: *Did you pick your career based on the proposed salary? Do you have any regrets now? If you could tell you 18-year-old self one thing about picking a career, what would it be?*

CHAPTER 11

Damned If I do. Damned If I don't.

"I am not interested in trying to convince and change the mind of a bigot."

—Angela Rye

Be excited, but not too excited. Be aggressive, but not overly aggressive. Show enthusiasm but don't overdo it. This is the advice we are inundated with in medical school. As a matter of fact, I would bet that many of us have heard this advice across multiple fields and not just medicine. We understand that there is a thin line between doing just enough and doing too much. The unfortunate truth is that as a minority, this line is even thinner. We must walk the tightrope with an added layer of cautiousness.

"Tamika, during your month on our service and during your interview day, many folks were impacted negatively. Some used the descriptor 'chip on her shoulder' and others the metaphor 'attitude'. Over a month of regular contact, that self-presentation softened. However during brief interviews, it left a strong negative impression. I cannot further explain the affect and certainly am not able to suggest its etiology nor management. Attitude is what we meant when we said we were looking for persons who were a good fit. Your affect and our expectations did not marry."

These are the words that were sent to me via email almost 10 years ago, and is still sitting in my inbox to this day. I received this email from a faculty member at a residency program that I did an elective month at in my last year of medical school, and interviewed at as a possible contender for my residency choices. Needless to say, I did not go to that program.

As students near the end of medical school, they have to choose what specialty they are going into. At the beginning of your 4th year, you apply widely to residency programs you are interested in across the country. In the fall, you begin to receive interviews with various programs. At the end of the interview season, typically in February of your last year, you have to submit a rank list. A rank list is where you list, in order of preference, the schools you interviewed at. If you did not receive an interview from a program, you are not allowed to rank them. On the other hand, just because you interviewed at a program does not mean that you have to rank them. Any program you rank, there is a possibility that you may end up there even if they are at the bottom of your list. Most mentors recommend ranking at least 10 programs, if possible, to ensure you have cast a wide enough net.

You submit this list to an electronic database. At the same time, every residency program has to rank applicants they interviewed. They cannot rank an applicant if they did not interview them. Typically, many OB programs receive thousands of applications, only extend maybe 100 interviews or less, and rank about 50 applicants. It's a very competitive process. They enter their list into this same online database. This database has a programmed algorithm to match candidates with residency programs. I always refer to it as "The Draft" for doctors. For example, if I rank a program number 1 and they rank me number 1, we will match. If I rank a program number 2 and they ranked me number 3 and they have 5 available slots, I would still match there, so long as my first choice did not rank me at the top of their list. As you can see, when there's thousands of applicants and hundreds of programs, the algorithm can get quite complicated, so you truly never know where you will end up.

Fast forward to a month later; in March there is a special day for all medical students called "Match Day". This is the day that medical students all over find out what residency program they "matched" into, if they matched at all. On Monday you receive an email late morning that says either "congratulations you matched" or "we regret to inform you that you did not match". For those students who matched, the following Friday is Match Day and you open up a sealed envelope to find out where you will be spending the next 3 to 7 years of your life. For those students who did not match, they have to try and "scramble" into one of the unfilled positions in the country.

The unfilled position could be at a program they have visited before, or it could be a program foreign to them. The unfilled position could also be in a completely different field. So essentially you can go to medical school for 4 years with your heart set on being a plastic surgeon in California, not match, and end up scrambling into an open position as a pathologist in New York. Crazy and stressful, right? You can also opt to wait another year and enter the interview process and match again in hopes of getting that plastic surgery spot in California. Many students prefer to match into SOMETHING rather than waiting a year, but several students would rather wait. It all depends on their desire and financial situation. Waiting a year may not sound too bad, but trying to find a job during that year can be difficult. You cannot work as a doctor, because you have not completed the residency training. You cannot work in many other positions that you may be labeled as "over-qualified" for. It's an uncomfortable limbo space to be in so the decision of how to proceed varies from person to person. Nonetheless, that is how 4th year of medical school is structured.

In the late summer and fall of your 4th year, while you are waiting on interview requests to roll in, you have the option of doing an "away rotation". Built into our curriculum, are electives and you can opt to do those at your home school or visit another medical school and do your elective. Many students use this as an opportunity to visit a program they are interested in. It gives you additional exposure to that field, with a little bit more autonomy than you had as a third-year medical student. You are supposed to function on the level as an intern.

The rotations are typically a month long and expectations are high. Due to the length and high stakes, some mentors recommend that students do not do an elective at one of their top choices for residency. If anything less than favorable happens, it could hurt your chances of matching there. Let's face it, that's easy to do for a medical student who is brand new to the system who is being scrutinized with every breath they take. Other mentors recommend going to one of your top choices to really shine and increase your chances of matching there. However, they do warn students, and I wholeheartedly agree, that this is essentially a month-long interview. With that being said, students are advised to put their best foot forward; be on time, be friendly, be professional at all times, help everyone out, be enthusiastic, and possibly kiss a little ass.

While this month-long interview can truly increase your chances of matching there, it also helps the student to know the program better. It is quite possible you thought you loved a program, and you get there and it is not a good fit. Or you think you would love living in Utah, and then after spending a month there, you realize it's boring and you would hate to be stuck there for the next 3 to 7 years of your life. I always advise my mentees to make the best decision for them and it truly varies from person to person. For some students, it could be career suicide and for others, it can help to overcompensate for a lower GPA or board scores.

Ok, so now you understand the structure and purpose behind an away rotation. So that excerpt from an email above is what I received from Dr. Strite—the doctor I worked with on my first away rotation. I actually haven't shared those hurtful words with anyone except my parents until now. When I read that email, I was devastated. Although that program was not my first choice, it was a program I was considering ranking. I spent a month with the doctor, in his private office, who wrote that to me. What's funny is that I felt a completely different vibe. There were two doctors that worked in that office and no residents or students alongside me, so I would gain a front row seat to all of the procedures and clinic visits that month. I was excited. One of the doctors, Dr. Berg was super friendly and he used much of his free time in between patients to speak with me about the field. Unfortunately, he went on medical leave very early in the month so I never saw him again. I spent the remainder of the month with just one doctor, Dr. Strite and his office staff.

I showed up early every day, read up on relevant topics every night, was friendly to everyone in the office, asked appropriate questions, and was hungry for more. He seemed to enjoy my company, and even invited me to after hours journal clubs and dinners as his guest. I enthusiastically attended, even though it was not a requirement for my rotation. Not once did he mention anything about my behavior or "attitude" and as good as I am in reading people, I never got a negative vibe from him at all. I thought the month went well. At my interview, I interacted with more people at the dinner as well as in the hospital. Everyone seemed friendly and down to earth. I was a bit shy, as I was nervous during every interview, but that is to be expected. I still went out of my way and came out of my shell to start conversation with everyone.

Receiving an email shortly after I sent an email thanking them for their time and such an awesome experience definitely had me perplexed. *A chip on my shoulder? Attitude?* I didn't understand. Reading further into the email, he said that my "self-presentation softened" during the month. *Was it harsh and rough initially? What was so aggressive and rough about my presentation?* I couldn't help but to think it had something to do with me being a Black woman. Now of course I cannot verify the underlying meaning behind this email, but I will tell you that it went on to essentially recommend that I do not rank their program as I was not wanted there.

More often than not, Black women are described using these words even before we open our mouth. We are commonly seen as intimidating and strong and angry as opposed to passive and dainty and friendly. Because of this truth, Black women find themselves in this awkward space between speaking up, demanding respect, or quietly ignoring microaggressions to avoid being labeled or Blackballed. When it comes to negotiations with our employers, Black women find it to be very difficult. We want to demand the salary we know we are worth but do not want to be perceived as combative. We want to speak out about the sexual harassment at the job but do not want to be perceived as a troublemaker. We want to be addressed by the same titles as everyone else with our credentials rather than "baby" or "sweetie", but we do not want to be perceived as the complainer.

There's a very fine line and we understand this more than anyone else and because of that, we have to pick a lane and ride it out for the journey. I think timing is key. To climb the ladder of success, its necessary to humbly let a lot of shit go. I am not saying to allow disrespect by any means; however, picking your battles is essential. To me, it's just like softball—you don't swing at every ball, but you wait for the pitcher to throw you a good ball then you hit it as hard as you can. If you swing at every ball, especially the low ones, you may strike out when in actuality, you may have been given a base after so many balls from the pitcher. As you make your way to the top of the ladder, you have more room to make your demands known and use your voice. You will then have the opportunity to speak for those without a voice, as you once were. At that point, you could still be labeled many things and frowned upon, but when you've positioned yourself in a place of power, you get to call the shots.

When I received that email, I cried like a baby. I was crushed to my core. I worked hard, spent countless amounts of hours with this doctor, including time after work in my free time in efforts to show how interested and eager to learn I was and it wasn't enough. I was discouraged; especially to receive that in the middle of the interview cycle. I read it to my mom over and over again and she was so upset because she watched how hard I had worked that month and she knew firsthand, what was going on and how I felt.

I wrote a lengthy, yet professional response back. There was a lot of emotion being felt at the time so I saved it as a draft and came back to it when I gathered myself. I highly recommend that to everyone. Never send an email at the height of your emotion. I edited it here and there and once it was perfect, I was ready to send it. That draft has been sitting in my inbox for almost a decade. I never sent it. I thought long and hard about it. I prayed about it. While I do not know if he sent that personally or if anyone in the program even knew he sent that to me, it was a reflection of the program and I did not want to go to a program that felt that way about me. Despite it being against the rules to send an email like that to an applicant saying "do not rank us, because we won't be picking you," I did not escalate that matter at all. I did not qualify it with a response at all and I never spoke to nor ever crossed paths with Dr. Strite again.

When I speak about picking ones' battles, this was one I chose to let go. God had major plans in store for me, my life, and my career, and this was an affirmation that His plans were not to send me there. Now, almost 10 years later, I can say for certain that everything worked out the way it was supposed to and I ended up taking the path that was designed for me. I learned a valuable lesson here.

Although I did not feel I had any negative interactions with him or this "chip on my shoulder" as he described, it did make me take a second look at my body language and non-verbal communication. I also made an effort to smile more and attempt to soften my appearance. You can say that I should not have changed anything and been true to myself, but honestly I felt being true to myself was digging deeper and seeing how I was going to grow from this negative encounter. I wanted to see what could I take away from it.

This encounter has allowed me to be a better mentor. I make sure my mentees are cognizant of their non-verbal communication and that a little goes a long way. Although I am never going to encourage anyone to kiss ass, or be someone that they aren't, sometimes you do have to play the game. By playing the game, I mean smiling a bit more, seem a little more interested in your colleague's daughter's 4th birthday party, and attempting to be social by grabbing lunch or a drink after work sparingly with the team. It may seem like a "damned if I do, and damned if I don't" situation, but I've learned that the smallest things that take little to no energy on your part can make the world of a difference on how others perceive you, especially if you're a minority. Play the game until you are in a position to create your own game.

Affirmation to recite: *I will remain humble. When I climb the ladder of success, I will be sure to use my platform to help others that do not yet have their own.*

Question: *When was a time that you experienced a negative situation, but decided to ignore it and not react nor respond? What made you decide to ignore it? Do you regret not speaking up? At this point in your life, would you respond differently?*

Part IV

The Emergence (Residency)

CHAPTER 12

Faith the Size of a Mustard Seed

"You wanna fly, you got to give up the shit that weighs you down."

—Toni Morrison

On March 15, 2013, I matched into OBGYN specialty at a program in Ohio. Although this was not my first choice, it was in the top three. I had spent four of the roughest years of my life away from family and friends and I wanted to be close to home again. Toledo, Ohio is about an hour from Detroit and I knew I would be seeing my family frequently. I also loved the residency program director and her husband who both ran the program. They both were great mentors, surgeons, and overall awesome people with great morals. They were tough on us and I always gravitated towards mentors like that. It's like the love-hate relationship between an athlete and his or her personal trainer or coach.

When I arrived on the first day of orientation, I saw that the campus and program lacked diversity. I wasn't shocked, but it was a small adjustment coming from spending the last four years at a Historically Black College and University (HBCU) for medical school. Being the only Black female doctor in the program, I knew there would be some obstacles, but I was so excited to be a doctor that the rest would breeze past me—or so I thought. Upon meeting my classmates, I saw who I would likely befriend and who I likely would not. But my naiveté did not allow me to foresee the bullshit that was in my near future.

I did not realize the huge rift between some of the physicians in the program. In actuality, it was between the two hospitals that we rotated at. The community hospital and the university hospital. The doctors and staff of one did not get along with the doctors and staff of the other. The residents who had to spend time at each place frequently assumed the role of the "redheaded stepchild" smack in the middle. It was all pretty juvenile, if you ask me. The residents ended up taking sides and perpetuating gossip. I got along with everyone and did not really care about the historical rifts. I just wanted to become an OBGYN. I frequently went home to be with my family and friends or watch Michigan football games that Fall. The drama got so bad that I unknowingly got pushed right into the middle with everyone else.

One of my classmates, Kelsey, was the prototypical "fake friend". She would smile in your face and talk about how much she wanted to help you then turn around and talk about you like a dog. I remember one time, I was drowning with my notes, consults, etc. All of my classmates started off at this hospital and learned the system together. I was placed at a different hospital for my first month. So when I came to the community hospital in my second month, they had the hang of things logistically and it was like day one for me being that I had never stepped foot in there before.

She offered to help me get my notes done and show me how things were done there. I remember being so appreciative. Thinking, thank God Kelsey is here to show me around and how they like stuff done at this hospital. Well that little witch went and told my attending (our supervising physician) that she was doing all the work, and I was struggling terribly. This was one of many incidents that her conniving, misguided, low self-esteem tail was involved in. She befriended some of the upper-level residents, chiefs, and attendings and had them eating out the palm of her hand. Intern year is hard. Your first year being a doctor, in a new place, learning how to handle this new responsibility and getting your bearings, will of course be quite bumpy. Kelsey added the extra drama that made intern year terrible. She was in the middle of every personal and professional scandal and drama and talked about everyone. She had a special hate for me though. It showed through her continued betrayal and attacks. I never did anything to her and I learned to accept that she was jealous and intimidated by this smart Black doctor from Detroit.

Despite her harassing me all year long, lying to attendings, and painting the picture that she was the hardest worker, I kept to myself and kept pushing. This girl wasn't going to deter me from my goal that I worked my butt off a lifetime for. I became immune to it. They can think what they want about me, but one thing is for sure: my work ethic is impeccable and I genuinely care about my patients. The day intern year that I was brought to tears was the day that my work ethic was questioned.

One of my new younger attendings who befriended my kiss ass classmate Kelsey, was constantly picking on me. It was not the same kind of picking on when someone sees potential and wants to push you further. It was a berating, genuine dislike, and disrespectful kind of picking. I pulled her aside one day and asked if we could talk in her office. She agreed. When I asked her why she was so ugly to me day in and day out despite what I do, her response had me in tears. I think I had a ray of hope that this was just in my head and she liked me and wanted to push me to my potential. She told me, "Tamika I think you are lazy. You are not a hard worker and you cut corners. I see your classmate doing so much more than you. So yeah I don't like people who are lazy."

Wow. I had never in the 25 years of my life been called lazy before. To have a supervising physician who had been working with me for just a month call out my work ethic and summarize me as the lazy Black girl was heartbreaking. She did not see behind the scenes. She did not know that I was coming to work at 4 AM before everyone else and prepping notes and seeing patients. I worked quietly. Kelsey made sure she had an audience when she did things.

All these things I considered explaining, but I knew what type of person she was. She was the type of person who had already made up her mind about me and it wasn't my job or desire to try to change it. I wiped my tears and told her "I am sorry you feel that way about me, but you're furthest from the truth." I remember talking to my program director about the encounter and she assured me that she knew exactly how hard of a worker I was and not to let that throw me off my tracks. I held onto her words as I navigated through the remainder of the year. Never let someone's words define you. You know who you are and as long as you hold tight to that, you will never lose your way.

I frequently had to stop in patients' doorways to show my badge because I was not believed to be the physician. I had patients and their families asking me left and right if I had finished high school. I had one patient that waited until I had finished checking her cervix then asked me "Next time you check me can you put gloves on?" Seriously? Why would I examine anyone's vagina without wearing gloves? The nurse chuckled and reassured the patient that I had gloves on for the exam. The nurse went on to explain the gloves were a special type and beige/brownish color. The patient laughed and responded "I've seen those gloves before, I guess I have never had a doctor that matched those gloves though. I thought it was just her skin!" The room was full of laughter.

What's funny? I had so many encounters and situations during my intern year that it made me want to quit several times. I felt that if I quit, I would be letting myself down and letting "my people" down. *I am the only Black female doctor in the program, if I quit, what message will that send about the next Black girl that tried to come here? I had to keep pushing.*

One of the fourth-year residents who was also "Team Kelsey" and a complete witch herself, Sherry, gave me a hard time as well. She did the same fake smiles, lies behind your back, etc. She was someone I avoided at all costs when I could. But since she was a fourth year and I was a first year, I had to follow her orders when we worked together. She also singled me out and treated me worse than anyone in the program. I started seeing a pattern. Why me? I did not do anything to anyone. I did not talk about anyone. I went to work, came home, and did it again.

Well at the end of the year in a residency meeting, people were expressing their concerns and issues out loud. I was quiet. At this point I did not care and was completely desensitized to it all. My friend and classmate Ana expressed her concern for how Sherry treated residents and then pointed to me as an example. She explained that Sherry was targeting me for no reason and I didn't deserve it. I was so surprised and it caught me off guard. Sherry began crying and explaining that she had been stuck by a needle during surgery on an HIV patient and was on anti-HIV drugs (routine protocol with needlestick injuries) and that they were making her behave that way toward me. She apologized in front of everyone for giving me such a rough year and came over to hug me. I didn't move from my chair. The tears were real. The apology was not.

It was almost comical, honestly. I wanted to ask her, "Sherry, what anti- HIV drugs have 'being a bitch to the Black girl in the program' as a side effect?", but instead I smiled and stayed in my seat. She wasn't worth the debate, nor the energy. Again, it's all about choosing your battles. You may think of a million clapbacks during times of adversity, but taking the high route is important. It speaks to your professionalism and character. Like Michelle Obama said, "when they go low, we go high". I say this over and over in my head every time I want to clap back with a witty comment. And boy oh boy, do I have a million in queue. It's not worth it. Bite your tongue and keep it moving!

Now don't get me wrong, everything was not dreadful about Toledo. Most of the private doctors, attendings, and midwives were awesome, and the nurses were super helpful and sweet. They made the experience so much better when I was in my moments of wanting to quit. Also, one of my classmates Ana and I became really close friends. She along with a few upper-level residents like Amy and Veronica became friends who I still keep in touch with to this day.

I knew intern year was going to be rough. I had heard that from everyone who had come before me. But I honestly began to feel that I was going through a little more than the normal. From the racism, not being a good fit, to the drama with the program and a mass exodus of our leadership in our program, something did not feel right. I did what any

Christian would do in a conflicted situation, I prayed about it. God told me my time there was up and I needed to leave. As much as I wanted His approval to quit, I was scared to quit. I worked so hard to get here, and I was trying to prove that this little Black girl from Detroit was truly smart and strong and could endure anything.

That's when I had to learn, dear reader, you cannot make everyone appreciate or respect your greatness. No matter what I did or how long I stayed, the people who were making it so difficult for me for whatever reason were never going to change how they viewed me. I could beg, bake them muffins, and give them foot massages like I saw others doing, but for what purpose? So why waste my time trying to prove that I can survive and that I am a nice, caring person and compassionate doctor, instead of moving on where I can flourish academically and personally? Do not feel obligated to stay in a situation that you are not able to grow in. The grass is always greener on the other side, as they say, so understand there will be struggles in both situations. I did not flee one situation hoping to come to a perfect program. I fled one situation hoping to be able to be in an environment conducive to learning OBGYN, instead of dealing with the insignificant personal scandals and marital affairs of colleagues. Be sure to make a decision that is best for you may it be personally or professionally, or often times, both. God told me this year was my last year in Toledo so I had to accept that, but I did not have a clue what to do.

I called up my OB mentor from Meharry, Dr. Byrd. I explained everything to her including the fact that only 7 months into residency, our program did not have a program director, assistant program director, department chair, medical student clerkship director, etc. She agreed that I needed to find another program. She explained that I could either quit and have to go through the match process again and start residency over, or I could finish my intern year, then transfer to another program that has a vacant second-year position and pick up where I left off. I had been through so much in those seven months, there was no way in hell that I was going to redo that anywhere. I wanted my seven months of hell to count toward my residency completion.

I knew coming in as a second year to a new program would be tough, but again, there was no way I was going to repeat intern year. I searched for vacant positions and there were three in the entire country for second-year positions. Although I was discouraged that I would probably not be one of the three selected, I applied for two of the positions. One position was back home in Michigan at Beaumont Hospital. The other position was at University of Texas at Houston, which was my number one choice when I initially went through the match in 2013. I knew this was no coincidence that the place I wanted to train at originally now had a second-year position vacant right after God told me that my time at Toledo was finished.

I interviewed at both positions. I knew I really wanted to go to Houston, I loved the program, had already seen it in person, and God told me that was where I needed to be. I was led there in 2013 which is why I was confused when I had not matched there. But little did I know I would be there just a year later.

My apartment lease was up at the end of June right when my intern year was at the end. They sent a notice in the mail saying that if I wanted to move out, I needed to give 60 days' notice, which was the end of April. At that time, I still did not have a signed offer from UT Houston. I knew that if I did not put in my 60 days immediately, then I would be stuck in that apartment I was in, but I also knew that if I put in my 60-day move out notice and did not get another job, then I would have nowhere to live for my second year of residency in Toledo.

I have had my struggles with faith and trusting God, but this by far had to have been the hardest at that point in my life. God told me I was going to get a position elsewhere and I would not be in Toledo after June, so I needed to trust Him and sign my move out notice. My mind kept psyching me out and trying to convince me this was not practical. My parents even told me that I should wait until I have a job offer to sign a move out notice. I took a leap of faith and signed the move out notice at the end of April. May 1st, I signed a contract from UT Houston for a second year of residency beginning July 1. God carried me through that! Whew!

The hard part was over, or so I thought. Well now I needed to tell my program that I would not be returning for my second year. There was so much chaos going on in the program at that time, that I honestly could have not told anyone and been just fine. I didn't feel that was the right thing to do. They were making schedules for the upcoming year and I felt that I needed to tell them. My former program director knew, as she had written my letter of recommendation, but she had already quit and had no ties to the program anymore. I needed to tell the staff and residents who were still there.

At the end of the "monumental" resident meeting I described earlier when Sherry cried and apologized to me for being a witch, I stood up and announced that I was leaving the program. Everyone was in shock. Most of them did not even know you could transfer residency programs. Some of them were pissed because now they would have an empty position to fill for the next year. I gave them two months to figure those details out, and I did not even have to give that.

Those couple of months were rough, they retaliated like there was no tomorrow. I was treated even worse and my vacation was taken away from me. It was comical to me. They were salty. I was leaving. So who really won? To make matters worse, five residents left that year including me. This was about thirty percent of the program. Even though one of the soon-to-be chiefs left before I did, I was still viewed as the "ring leader" who made everyone want to leave. I did not encourage anyone to leave, nor did I discuss it with anyone, including my friends. I just did what was best for me.

When I came to Houston, I never looked back. This lazy little Black girl from Detroit went on to excel in Houston, be elected Chief Resident, win several awards, and join the faculty at one of the top OBGYN programs in the country.

Affirmation to recite: *I trust God. I trust the process. I trust my intuition.*

Question: *Have you ever felt strongly about a decision you needed to make, not made it, and regretted it? What was your inhibition in going with your gut? Would you make a different decision today?*

CHAPTER 13

Doctor Bae

"If someone lacked decency or respect, I didn't allow that person to stay in my world."

—Gabrielle Union Wade

In today's dating world, online dating has become increasingly more popular. One third of all married couples meet online nowadays. For those of you who may not be familiar with how many dating apps work, let me give a quick rundown. You create a profile with a few of your best pictures along with some basic information about yourself including age, occupation, city of residence or hometown, education level, if you have children, etc. In addition, you usually include a few fun facts about yourself or answer a few questions and post those to your profile as well. Your profile gets added to a large database of dating profiles. When you begin searching for "dating prospects" you can set your search filters to narrow your search. Profiles start popping up on your phone. You have the choice to scroll through their profile and either "swipe right", meaning you like them, or "swipe left" meaning you'll pass. When the app identifies two people who both like each other, they notify you and you can begin conversing with them. There's different rules and variations depending on the site, but in a nutshell, that's online dating.

Ok so ladies, you come across the profile of a nice-looking man in your desired age group. You scroll to view his profile and find out that you both share similar hobbies, he seems personable and witty based on his description on his profile. You scroll to see his occupation and he is a physician. Swipe right? Um, duh! He is worth a shot, right? I know some of you will disagree to play devil's advocate, but you get the point. He seems like a nice guy with similar interests, he is attractive, and has a great job, right?

So what if the tables are turned? Guys, if you are seeing the same profile, of an attractive young lady and see that her occupation is a physician, is this a for sure swipe right? Or do you swipe left? Are you still interested? I'm sure many of you will have mixed responses, but I can tell you from my friends' and my anecdotal experiences, more guys are likely to see that as a turn off than the opposite. I am not throwing statistics at you to support this argument. I am just speaking about my experiences. Often times, successful women are viewed as a turn off based on negative stereotypes. Successful working women can sometimes be viewed as overbearing, arrogant, argumentative, male bashing feminists who throw their money in a man's face at every chance possible. I am sure there are some women who have done that before, but that stereotype is getting pretty old. We need to take a minute to understand why some women may behave that way or are just simply viewed that way.

This country has not historically been in favor of women holding any type of power for centuries on end. Women did not use to have a voice. They were expected to shut up, stay in the house, care for the children and household chores, and for their spouse when he returned home from a long day at work. So naturally in the 20th century when women joined the workplace, started getting more post-secondary education, were allowed to vote, and began holding positions of power, some people were not prepared for the shift about to take place. Even in these jobs, women were always at the bottom of the totem pole.

Even lower than all women, were women of color. Being a double minority, women of color receive less respect and less pay for equal job responsibilities. I wish this was merely a history lesson, but this is true even today as I write this book. We have made significant strides on women's rights, but there is more work to be done until equal pay and equal respect is obtained.

Ok, off my soapbox about women's rights...

Many people who hold onto traditional views of the household still feel the management of the chores and children are a task for women only. Due to many middle-class households requiring two incomes to sustain their financial obligations, both men and women are working. So if both parties are working 40-hour work weeks and coming home tired, is it still expected that the woman get dinner ready, get the kids cleaned up, and the house cleaned up too? Basically. In my generation, I see a lot of men bashing women who don't know how to cook and clean, but never stop to realize that in our generation, the upbringing is fairly comparable. Boys and girls are both going to school, then getting jobs after graduating, and so on. Home economics courses are rarely a part of the school curriculum in this day and age. So when are girls learning these "womanly duties"? In their spare time?

Nonetheless, I'm not going to focus on the myriad views I have heard over the years, nor even express my own. I was just simply outlining some of the contradictory thought processes that many of us harbor. We cannot simply expect a woman to do the same duties as a man, receive no respect, less pay, then expect them to come home and take care of everyone in the household but themselves and then wonder why our women are dying from preventable diseases and stress. Not just women who do not have access to healthcare due to finances, but women who do have access but they put everyone and everything before themselves. I take care of women for a living. It's my reality. I see it every single day. Women are going decades without PAP smears and mammograms, which are essential screening tests for preventing and catching early stage cancers.

So after considering all the things mentioned that women are enduring, with women of color enduring the most disrespect and inequalities, maybe we can see where the title "angry Black woman" came from. Are we angry, or just tired of the disrespect, unequal pay, lack of appreciation and bullshit? In order to navigate the rollercoaster life throws at us, women must develop skin thick enough to weather the harshest of the storms. This thick skin is what helps us demand our power and respect, and climb the ladder of success in obtaining our well-deserved accolades. Unfortunately, the same thick skin we have used to become successful, is the same thick skin that can label us "undateable". Now ladies, just because you are successful and established, this does not give you a pass to belittle and emasculate every man that tries to approach you. He does not need to hear about your résumé and how independent you are and that you don't need a man for anything. These all may be great attributes, but boasting for the mere purpose of putting down your partner is not ok.

The double standard can be frustrating. Why is it that a successful strong man is looked at as a hot commodity in the dating world, but a successful strong woman is perceived as the danger zone? Of course not everyone shares these views, but there are enough out there who do, or else I would not have a chapter worth of information to write about. While I was in medical school, I would watch our male classmates interact with women when we would all go out. They would almost always slide in the line "I am about to be a doctor" at every introduction. I cannot knock them for it. The ladies loved it, so it worked. Then on the other hand, I would watch female classmates wait until several dates in to drop the "bomb" that she is in school to be a doctor. Many of us were hiding under some general job title. I routinely used "I am in the medical field" and let them assume I was a nurse or medical assistant like they always do anyways. I know, that sounds egregious right? I wish I was lying, but these are facts! We learned early on that we would scare many guys away by the mere fact that we were soon-to-be physicians.

This continued even past school and well into my career. I always paused when asked what I did for a living. I purposely avoided asking men what they did, in fear that they would reciprocate the question. You may be reading this and think I am crazy. But I know I am not alone. I also know that this does not just apply to physicians and there are many other successful strong women who have battled the same insecurity. The bigger question is why is this an insecurity? Something you work so hard to achieve and put in countless amounts of hours and sacrifice and now you're "hiding it" rather than being proud. I wish I could say this did not apply to me, but it definitely does and I know this battle all too well, unfortunately.

I remember speaking to my girlfriends about it one day and they were appalled. They could not believe that I was out here "acting ashamed" of my hard-earned profession. I did not feel that I was ashamed of it at all, but I can see why they said that. Why was I feeling the need to dilute my success in hopes of finding a good man? The kind of man I wanted would not be insecure over the fact that I am a doctor and I knew that, but it honestly was a hard habit for me to break. We must all move past these silly nuances and just be proud that we are all achieving great things. Women, if a man is intimidated by your success, he likely is not the one for you. On that same token, I definitely think we can sometimes do a better job at not throwing our résumé and salary out at every chance we get. They get it! You worked hard for it! That job isn't going to keep you warm at night though...

Another hurdle I have noticed in dating as a professional woman, is time commitment. Obviously with the success comes the time commitment one must put in to get there and stay there. Cancelled dates, postponed trips, late nights at school or work are all a part of the recipe for success. I personally felt that even after climbing the hurdles to find a good relationship, it was just as hard to maintain one. I am not a cheater, and never have been. I wish I had a dollar for every time I was accused of lying or cheating due to my crazy school or work schedule. I get it. It sounds real suspect that you're coming home in the middle of the night, going in super early, etc. I have been told things like "you're not feminine enough" or "you're not passive enough to be any man's wife" or "what do you need a man for if you can do everything for yourself?"

For many years I would cringe when thinking back to the men who said things like that to me. I one day stopped and tried to dissect what they were saying. Although the words may not have been put together in the best way, I was eventually able to learn about myself through those comments. I've never been the "damsel in distress" type of woman, and I enjoy watching sports in my free time. That's who I am, but that does not make me any less feminine than the next woman. One guy told me that he got upset when he came to my apartment to help me put my furniture together only to find that I knew my way around the toolbox better than he did. My dad was very handy and being a daddy's girl growing up, I learned a thing or two and became pretty resourceful myself. Not to mention, both of my parents worked in construction for the majority of my life.

Was this really about me not being feminine or was it his own insecurity about not being as handy as he would have liked? In hindsight, I guess I could have let him put together a few bookshelves or something. He just wanted to feel needed and it took me some years to realize that.

The guy who told me I wasn't passive enough to be a wife was not a fan of my voice. I have always been relatively outspoken with issues I am passionate about. I did not see how that would make me a bad wife. I just was not meant to be *his* wife, because he wanted a quiet, passive, "yes" girl. That wasn't me and still isn't today. I challenge people to think outside the box. I have a witty rebuttal for almost everything, which has gotten me into trouble a time or two (or three) in the past. I am not going to just agree with you if I think it's a bad idea. I have a brain and can form my own opinions.

With that being said, if you decide to pursue something and you're passionate about it, I am going to support my man through it all, regardless of how I feel. To me, that's more important than agreeing with everything a man says. If you ask me my opinion, I am going to give it. But if you don't, I don't necessarily need to be outspoken with my opinion. Knowing when and how to voice your opinion is crucial in a relationship. It makes the difference in coming off as supportive versus a negative Nancy. So again, I was able to take this negative comment and learn something about myself from it to apply to my future. That's what matters.

One guy I dated was super supportive at first. He said he loved the fact that I was a doctor and didn't understand why any man would be intimidated by that. He was fun to hang around, our dates would last for several hours, and we always enjoyed a good laugh. He worked in a plant and made great money. He loved his job and never seemed ashamed to come over or meet up with me in public with his work jumpsuit on. Everything was going well.

Shortly after I finished residency, I took some time off to relax and travel. I counted down the days of the end of my residency because I truly needed a break before starting my first official job as an attending physician. The only issue with taking time off before starting work, is that you're not getting a paycheck. With making a minimal amount of money in residency and spending much of it on applications, interviews, and travel, I didn't exactly have a ton of money stacked up in my savings account.

Money was tight and grew tighter. I also had sold my house, but the new house I had under contract was found to have over $50,000 in damages from Hurricane Harvey. The seller of the house was sneaky and painted over mold and discoloration. Luckily, I had a great inspector who noticed that something wasn't right and recommended I had a stucco inspector drill holes into the wall to assess the wood underneath. Although it was another cost during a time I made no income at all, it saved me from further headaches and heavy bill in the long run. I was going to have to rebuild half of the house due to rotting wood underneath the spongy stucco material.

The house was a European style, flat-top roof and was not built with metal caps to protect the stucco. So after torrential rain for 6 days with Hurricane Harvey, all the water seeped into the porous stucco and caused the wood to rot. I had to back out of the contract during the option period. I was relieved and panicking at the same time because I sold my house and had nowhere to stay. I was able to stay in my house a little bit longer and pay the new buyer's rent, but it got to a point where they were ready to move into their new home, and I couldn't blame them. I was stressed out.

I communicated what was going on to the guy I was dating. He was always so supportive and knew what to do. He comforted me and was supportive and trying to help me find an apartment that I could move in to within days. I hated this time of stress as I have always been a planner. I was thankful to have a supportive person in my life to help me.

I remember around that same time, Gabrielle Union had just come out with her first book, and as a huge fan of hers for several years, I was one of the first to grab her book. I was reading it in my spare time and I was locked in because it was so good, so raw, so real, and it made me love her even more for sharing so much of her life and experiences with the world. I was shocked to come across my name in her book! She referenced my story when I had gone viral for being barred from assisting an unresponsive passenger on a plane because the flight crew didn't believe I was a doctor.

The story was all over the news, magazines, internet, etc. She referenced my story in her book, unbeknownst to me, to parallel it to what her experience was as a Black actress in Hollywood. She had undergone the same type of discrimination. At a time where I was so overwhelmed and emotional about the many stressors in my life with money, housing, etc., seeing my name in the memoir written by one of my favorite actresses instantly had me in a good mood. As people started reading her book more and more, friends and family kept texting and calling me informing me that my name was written in her book. One of my friends tagged me on social media with a picture of my name in her book. I shared it on my timeline explaining how excited I was.

My beau came over after work that day and had seen my social media post.

"Tamika, I see you had a great day huh? I saw about Gabrielle Union mentioning you in her book," he chuckled.

"Yes babe, isn't that crazy? You know how much I love her! I am so excited!" I exclaimed.

He paused.

"Social media is such a façade. Especially people like you," he said.

"What does that mean?" I snapped back. He seemed irritated and I didn't understand where this was coming from.

"I mean, you always post positive things on social media. You post only good stuff!" He said.

"Well what am I supposed to post on social media? Depressing things? Negative energy? I don't use social media as a diary. I post things that I like, want to share, or uplifting things for other people. Did you have a bad day at work? What's good?" I asked.

"I mean, looking at your social media, you seemingly have a perfect life. You passed your boards, you have a new job as assistant professor, Gabrielle Union mentioned you in her new book, the list goes on. People only see the positive things. But in actuality, you're broke as hell, can barely pay your mortgage, your parents are having to help you out and are essentially homeless, desperately looking for a place to live," he said boldly.

"Wow." I was speechless. There I was thinking he was my biggest supporter, and he was a full-blown hater. Why did he care if I shared or didn't share every single struggle and negative thing that happened to me on social media? I share things that are uplifting and positive. Where did all of this come from?

After cooling down, we sat down and had a conversation. This conversation revealed all of his insecurities. He didn't want to settle down anymore until he got a master's degree. He wanted to keep "dating" until he achieved that and was closer to my level. Where was this coming from? He revealed a lot of his inner feelings about the differences in our lives and jobs, with me being a doctor and him being a blue collar worker. I didn't care about those things, but he was so caught up in it. Needless to say, we ended up parting ways, but it literally came out of left field to me.

He did a great job at hiding how he felt and it was almost like he enjoyed watching me sweat and struggle. Even in my small moment of joy during such a stressful time, he was salty. I am not saying all men are that way, because they definitely are not. But it does take a secure man, who knows his worth and what he brings to the table, to date someone who may make more money than him. So many of us get caught up on status and salary, that it's hard to look beyond those things. When I look for a man who is equally yoked, it's not about finances. It's the intellect for me! Ha! But seriously, I care more about intellectual stimulation, ability to carry a good conversation, his willingness and ableness to be a provider and lead his family through following God, and someone who I respect, and equally respects me, honors me, and is fun to be around. As cliché as it sounds, money and the status are not the only things to everyone. Men, stop counting yourself out or feeling like a potential mate is out of your league based on material things. You can bring so much more to the table than a paycheck, so stop limiting yourself.

Dating a doctor is certainly not for the fainthearted, and I have so much respect for those who are able to sit tight for the long journey ahead. Dating a female doctor may present uncomfortable situations, or inappropriate jokes, or comments from friends or coworkers. At the end of the day, do you care what other people think or say? I honestly found it more exhausting having to deal with the stressors at school or work and then come home to try and maintain a relationship. I saw many successful relationships flourish and I have nothing but respect for them. I also saw many failed relationships for this very reason. I think having a stable relationship is a blessing and a curse. It's nice to have someone to vent to, spend time with outside of work, share some of the house duties with (unless you have one of those men I spoke about previously that wouldn't dare touch a dirty dish). I can also see how difficult it is to split time between personal and work and not have either party feel slighted. This ends up making the person (woman or man) feel drained from trying to please everyone.

I have had times where I regretted not putting more effort and sacrifices into making certain relationships work, and other times where I have regretted the wasted time and energy put into a relationship rather than school or work. Over time, I realized that I learned a lot about myself through those situations and I should never regret things that helped make me who I am. It's all about making the right choices at the right time. Unfortunately, we aren't always privy to that beforehand and it ends up being a trial and error type of situation. I regularly tell myself, "Win some. Lose some. Learn from all. Regret none." At the end of the day, everyone has to do what is best for them and just understand that the grass isn't always greener on the other side. Trying to see things from your partner's perspective is key if you're trying to make a relationship work.

> ***Affirmation to recite***: *I will not dismiss my own success in an effort to make someone else feel more secure about theirs, or lack thereof.*

> **Question**: *When was a time that you felt your profession interfered with your relationship? What aspects of your profession interfered? Have you made any changes to prevent this from recurring in the future?*

CHAPTER 14

I Can't Breathe

"Young people are enraged. And there's an easy way to stop it. Arrest the cops. Charge the cops. Charge all the cops. Not just some of them. Not just here in Minneapolis. Charge them in every city across America where our people are being murdered."

—Tamika Mallory

The date was July 5th, 2016, and another hot Texas July 4th weekend had passed. To me, July 4th means barbecues, family gatherings, pool parties with friends, frozen drinks, and fireworks. I have many great July 4th memories growing up back home. In Detroit, our winters were cold and ugly but our summers were beautiful. Perfect weather for a solid three months was bliss to us Michiganders. As kids, we were out of school for the summer so we always had fun linking up with friends during this holiday weekend, or going on family vacations. That's what July 4th meant to me. So now, whenever I have the weekend off, I enjoy spending time with loved ones and keeping those traditions going.

To many Americans, the July 4th holiday, widely referenced as Independence Day, was created to celebrate our independence as a nation. Many celebrations include fireworks, patriotic décor and clothing. Red, white, and blue cookies and cakes and slushies or snowcones. As I grew older and wiser, I realized this widespread celebration of independence was not equally shared by all of us. To be Black in America, we still weren't free. Frederick Douglass' speech, "What to the Slave is the Fourth of July?" outlined this very notion. We were still slaves and even after physical bondage, we still faced racial discrimination and brutality. So for a nation that we consider home, it's a slap in the face to see celebration of freedom that has not always been shared by all of us.

We weren't free on July 4th, 1776, and we aren't free today. The nation continued in widespread celebration of Independence Day on July 4th, 2016, but on July 5th, Black people were reminded yet again that this holiday was not for us.

July 5th, 2016 was the day that Alton Sterling was fatally shot by the police in Louisiana. The police received an anonymous report that there was a man outside of a convenience store selling CDs and he had a gun. The store owner did verify that although Sterling had a gun for protection, he was not the suspect causing any trouble. The police approached Sterling, tasered him to the ground, kneeling on his chest and leg. When an officer claimed he was concerned that Sterling was reaching for a gun, he fired 6 rounds in his chest, killing him instantly. Another senseless killing of a Black man at the hands of a police officer. The anger, the hurt, the tears, were all felt by the Black community. We were outraged and are continuously asking ourselves, "When will this stop?" Going back to work after the holiday weekend and this horrible event wasn't easy. Black coworkers were talking about the tragic event. Many of our non-Black counterparts were silent, and business was as usual.

The very next day, July 6th, 2016, in Minnesota, Philando Castile was fatally shot. He was in the car with his girlfriend and her 4-year-old daughter. Castile informed the officer that he had a firearm after being pulled over for a routine traffic stop. The officer told him not to pull it out and him and his girlfriend emphatically assured the officer that he was not going to. When one of the two officers felt scared that he would reach for it, he fired 5 rounds into Castile, killing him almost immediately. The officer was placed on paid administrative leave. So in less than 48 hours, we lost two precious Black men at the hands of police officers, and the living proof was all on video. I do not even have the words to describe the pain the Black community felt during that time.

Racial tensions were high. Parents were scared to leave their Black children's side for fear that it may be the last time they seem them alive. To be in Black in America, we experience racism—both overt and covert—bias, and profiling on a regular basis. Regardless of how many times we endure these painful experiences, it never makes the next experience any easier to overcome. The build up of the hatred felt in this country that we call home is indescribable. At work, our non-Black counterparts were still quiet. No discussion of the outrage or the injustice. Silence.

On July 7th, 2016, the very next day after Castile's murder, protests in Dallas became violent with five officers killed, and 11 wounded. The gunman who opened fire was killed soon after. These events were televised on the news and every TV I walked by in the hospital was turned to the breaking news. I was mentally and emotionally drained at that point. The day was only half over, the week was only half over, and so much had happened already. I walked into the physicians' lounge to grab my lunch. In walked another physician.

"Oh my God! Did you guys see what happened to the police officers in Dallas? Innocent police officers were just killed for no reason!"

Another physician added, "I know, it is so crazy and so sad! I cannot believe they are doing this to innocent people."

It took everything in me to keep my mouth shut and I could not resist another second.

"Yea, it is sad and unfortunate that innocent lives are being taken. Just like the two innocent Black men whose lives have been taken earlier this week! None of you mentioned anything about those incidents and now you want to discuss these police officers and you haven't said a damn thing all week. I'm disgusted," I announced.

My classmate walked into the lounge and heard my voice carrying. "What's going on? What's Cross talking about?"

"She's talking about race again," one physician blurted out with an annoyed facial expression.

My classmate turned to me and says, "Why are you so worked up anyways? They are killing Black men not Black women. Plus, you're light skinned anyways, I think you're safe," she smirked.

"My dad is a Black man, my brother is a Black man, my nephews will grow up to be Black men. I have grandparents, uncles, cousins, and close friends that are Black men. That's the most ignorant thing I've ever heard!" My anger was building up inside.

She stared at me blankly.

"Let's not forget about innocent Black women that have been killed too! Sandra Bland was literally killed damn near down the street from where we are standing right now!" I shouted back.

She responded flatly, "Sandra Bland? That's the girl who committed suicide. She doesn't count."

I grabbed my shit and left the lounge. I could not stomach another minute of this conversation.

That evening, I felt depleted. I had no emotional reserve. I was overwhelmed by the amount of hate being expressed daily, the senseless killing of our precious Black kings and queens, and the straw that broke the camel's back is debating with ignorant coworkers that will never understand the shoes that we walk in every single day. I called my brother and father on three-way that night. I was angry, I missed my family, I was scared for them, and most importantly, I wanted justice. They let me rattle off my emotions that ended in me crying like a baby. I was so damn tired.

For my own peace, I had to learn that if I wanted to avoid controversial conversations especially around topics that are emotionally arousing for me, I found it best to avoid common spaces such as the cafeteria or lounge. I have not walked into one of these common spaces at any job and not heard the discussion of religion, current events, politics, etc. For me personally, this was the only place we could keep our lunches and personal belongings so I had to frequent this common space. Many days I found myself eating in my call room, or in a hidden space for my mental peace and that was completely fine to me. Other days, it was inevitable to be in the physicians' lounge. I probably should have left the conversation earlier than I did, but I had no regrets with the exchange between us, but it left her still racist, and me even more emotionally drained.

I wish I could write this book as a fairytale and have a happy ending to share. I wish I could say that our nation took huge steps towards justice and that we are in a better place today. The killings of our Black kings and queens continued. Since July 2016, many more precious lives have been taken. Some received more media attention than others but that has nothing to do with the value of their lives and what they mean to us. DeAndre Ballard. Jamarion Robinson. Miles Hall. Botham Jean. Breonna Taylor. Ahmaud Arbery. Sean

Reed. George Floyd. David McAtee. Natosha McDade. The list has hundreds of names. This shit isn't getting any better.

On May 25, 2020, when George Floyd was murdered in cold blood by a police officer and the entire incident was recorded, the uproar of our nation got a bit louder. For over eight minutes, the video shows a white police officer kneeling on Floyd's neck while he gasped for air, pleading over and over again "I can't breathe". The world has heard those lasts words before with Eric Garner when he was killed by a police officer as well back in 2014. The graphic nature of this video has traumatized not only our Black community, but has begun to wake up those around us.

Despite being knee deep in one of the deadliest pandemics of all time, COVID-19, the country protested—some peaceful, some turned more violent—with riots breaking out all over the nation. This grotesque homicide of George Floyd was another heavy reminder that to this country, Black lives don't matter. So many people have an issue with the phrase "Black lives matter", feeling that it is ignoring other racial groups and that it is saying that they don't matter. I will never understand the narcissistic viewpoints of people who continue to believe that "Black lives matter" is offensive. It is purely a much needed reminder to a country that has shown us time and time again that Black lives don't matter.

How does one support that they feel Black lives matter while they kneel on a Black man's neck for eight minutes, while nonchalantly having your hands in your pockets and staring, unbothered, dead in the eyes of the camera man recording you? You feel that secure and that supported by a racist nation that you continue to press on despite Floyd's cry for help, cry for his mom, using his very last breaths to beg you for just another breath. Just as the other officers stood by, watching the life being taken from this Black man, are guilty for not speaking up against injustice, anyone in America that stands by and watches racist, discriminatory acts taking place around them, and is silent is just as guilty as well. Police brutality and injustice in America is not a "Black people problem" nor is it a "minority problem". It is our nation's problem and it is up to each and every one of us to do our part in fighting to fix a broken system.

What does it mean to be Black in America? It means that you are 2.5 times more likely to be killed by a police officer than a white person. It means that Black men between the age of 15 and 25 are nine times more likely to be killed by a police officer than any other race. Our ancestors marched and protested, fought, and died for injustice. Today we stand still fighting these same battles. While some may feel things will never change, I refuse to give up trying until we force these changes. Being Black in America is not easy, but if we ever want this country to be the place we imagined for our children and grandchildren, we must keep pressing on.

As a minority professional, we commonly find that our views are not shared by coworkers. What I find to be more disheartening is that despite the racial tensions experienced in this country, so many of our non-Black colleagues still do not understand nor care to understand what it is like to walk in our shoes. This is a recurring theme throughout school, training, and in my career so I am sure I am not alone. Make sure you have methods to unwind and decompress in a healthy fashion. It isn't about "if" you experience these things professionally, it is more about "when". Prepare yourself.

I don't think I will ever forget these tragic moments. The killings of our Black men and women seem to happen so frequently that one would think we would forget the specifics of a situation. As with any trauma, you remember specifics and you don't forget them. We all remember where we were on 9/11 and what we were doing. We remember the specifics on when tragic news of the loss of a loved one was delivered to you. These are traumatic events and science tells us that our brains will always make those associations.

To be Black in America, every senseless killing of our Black men and women is traumatic. We remember how we felt in those moments. We remember how people around us reacted in those moments. Those are things our brains can't erase. These are tragedies etched in our hearts forever, because every time another Black man or woman is killed, we all realize that it could have just as easily been one of us, and next time it may be.

Affirmation to recite: *I will continue to do what is right even if no one around me agrees or supports me.*

Question: *Can you recall a time when you felt uncomfortable in your workplace or when conversations got tense and your views were the minority? How did you feel? How did you react?*

CHAPTER 15

#Whatadoctorlookslike

"What I want young women and girls to know is that you are powerful and your voice matters."

—Vice President Kamala Harris

"Hey Tamika, my family is having a barbecue at my parents' house later on today to say a special thank you to all of my wedding party! This wedding weekend would not have been the same without all of you! Will you be able to come by or are you leaving town today?"

"Hey Britt, I am actually not leaving until Sunday, so I would love to come by. See you then!"

On October 8, 2016, these were the texts exchanged between my childhood friend, Brittany and me. I had just flown home for the week to stand by her side as a bridesmaid in her wedding. The ceremony and reception were beautiful and we all had a wonderful time celebrating their nuptials. Although her wedding was on a Friday, my flight out of Detroit did not leave until Sunday. That was pretty typical for my visits home; spend every possible second I could at home catching up with family and friends.

Later that day, I headed over to Brittany's parents' house for the barbecue and we had an amazing time. Just before I was heading out, I stopped in the living room to talk with her parents and oldest brother, Michael. Our families had known each other for many years and it always felt good to catch up face to face. We were discussing my job and how proud they were of me reaching my childhood dream of becoming a physician. I was explaining how much I loved what I did and although it was taxing, I did not regret one second of my journey.

As we wrapped up the conversation, I headed home to pack and prepare for my flight in the morning. I laid in bed that night reflecting on how much I miss home. Having lived out of state for the past seven plus years was difficult for a family oriented person like myself. I missed a lot of pivotal milestones: graduations, weddings, birthdays, holiday gatherings etc. Houston was where God led me and I felt was best for my career at that time, despite being several hundred miles away from home.

I woke up Sunday morning, October 9, 2016 and got my last-minute things together. The weather was chilly in Michigan, but I knew it would be warm in Houston (always my struggle trying to decide on plane attire when flying home). I decided it would be best to wear a sweatshirt as a compromise between the two climates. I threw on my Blue and Red "Detroit vs Everybody" sweatshirt, a pair of black leggings, my all black Toms, and headed out to the airport with my mom.

I boarded the flight, DL945, Zone 3, and toward the back of the plane on the right hand side. I always preferred a window seat, as it was better for napping. I unfortunately had an aisle seat on this leg of my flight from Detroit to Minneapolis, but I was comforted in knowing that when I changed planes in Minneapolis, I would have a window seat for that final leg to Houston. I decided I would watch a movie since I couldn't nap comfortably in my aisle seat.

Halfway through my movie, I thought I heard yelling, even with my headphones on. That is NEVER a good sign on a plane. I snatched off my headphones and confirmed there was in fact yelling. There was a woman who was two rows in front of me and on the left who was yelling stating that her husband was unconscious. A middle-aged flight attendant was already investigating the issue by time I had looked up. What was going on? Unconscious on a plane? Was he in a deep sleep? Did he need medical attention? All of these questions were running through my mind a million miles a minute. The flight attendant yells out, "Everyone calm down. He is alright. He just had a night terror. Everything is ok!" The other passengers all had expressions of relief on their face. I was still confused. Night terror made him unconscious? That's odd. I get back to watching my movie, but I left my headphones off as I still frequently glanced over at the couple, silently investigating. The flight attendant was still talking with the two of them.

Just a couple minutes later, it happened AGAIN. The poor man was unconscious again and this time the flight attendant began to panic. "Alright we need to call for a doctor or nurse or medical personnel overhead now!" she shouted to another flight attendant in the back of the plane as she begins to scurry back there as well. I immediately threw my tray table up and unbuckled my seatbelt to get up and assist when she was just passing my row. Rather than tapping/grabbing her as she was running past me, I raised my hand in effort to signal her attention (I have never been too keen on grabbing/touching strangers). She replied "Oh no sweetie, we need an actual physician or nurse or some type of medical personnel. We don't have time to talk to you!"

I repeatedly tried to inform her that I was a physician but she continued to cut me off with more condescending remarks. Did she think I was asking for a coke and Biscoff cookie? By this time, the other flight attendant was making the announcement on the PA system. "If there are any physicians on board, please press your call button!" I go to press my call button and the same flight attendant responds, "Oh wow, you're an actual physician?"

"Yes" I reply emphatically.

She began firing questions, "Let me see your credentials. Where do you work? What type of doctor are you? Why were you in Detroit?"

The unconscious passenger still has not been tended to.

I respond quickly, "OBGYN, work in Houston, in Detroit for a wedding, but believe it or not, they DO have doctors in Detroit. I do not have a badge or business card on me. Now excuse me so I can help the passenger."

Another middle-aged Caucasian male approached the scene from the front of the plane to help and stated he is a physician. The flight attendant turned to me and said, “Thanks for your help but he can help us and he has his credentials.” Mind blown. How did she know he had credentials? What makes him more fit to help than me? I stay seated as requested and continue to watch the scene. The other physician was asking questions and the man appeared to be responding. This is improvement. Thank God.

After about ten mins, the same flight attendant approached me and asks “What do you think we should do now, doc?” Wow, I have been upgraded from a sweetie to a doc! I explain that it is hard to say not knowing what was going on, but I would be sure to check vital signs and glucose. She came back with a piece of paper folded in half with “80/50” written on it and they cannot find a glucometer on board at all. We continued to discuss potential work up and she is personally relaying my words to the other physician (who is now sitting in the row with the couple). The other physician continued to sit with them for the remainder of the flight.

The same flight attendant kept approaching me and apologizing for the “mix up”. She made small talk with me about how she loves labor and delivery (since she learned I was an OBGYN) and how her daughter had delivered a baby recently. Needless to say, I was still in shock and not the least bit interested in the small talk. She asked me for my SkyMiles number, explaining that she wanted to give me SkyMiles for the mix up. I kindly refused. I had already made up my mind that I was reporting her and no amount of SkyMiles was going to quiet me from reporting blatant discrimination. Upon landing, the paramedics escorted the man off the plane as the rest of us passengers sat in our seats with feelings of relief that he was seemingly better.

When I finally deplaned, I went immediately to the gate front desk. I explained briefly the situation, and the gate agent directed me to Gate F1 where the "Need Help?" sign was. I went to that gate and asked for the Gate Manager. A middle-aged man of color greeted me and listened to my complaint. I explained that this was an emergency and proper protocol was not followed and the outcome could have been very different. He expressed his disgust with the situation. He encouraged me to fill out the Delta Online Survey then handed me a free drink ticket for my troubles. While it was obvious he was genuinely sorry and trying to comfort me, I felt this was completely inappropriate. This could have cost a passenger his/her life and you think a free rum and coke will solve the issue? If no one was going to take me serious here, I knew I had to take things higher. I walked to my next gate for my flight from Minneapolis to Houston. As I sat down waiting to board this flight, I was on the phone with my mother venting about the situation. My mom was infuriated and the more she saw how upset I was, the more upset she got, trying to find a way to console me. She is my mother, so she knows how persistent I am when passionate about something. She knew I was not going to rest until someone at Delta properly addressed this concern and heard me out. After all, I am a doctor and my job is to problem solve. I identified a major problem and needed a resolution to happen. I explained that no one seemed to care about this serious safety concern. Out of sheer frustration, I typed the what soon became "infamous Facebook post" sitting there at the gate waiting to board my next flight.

It read:

> "I'm sure many of my fellow young, corporate America working women of color can all understand my frustration when I say I'm sick of being disrespected. Was on Delta flight DL945 and someone two rows in front of me was screaming for help. Her husband was unresponsive. I naturally jumped into doctor mode as no one else was getting up. Unbuckled my seatbelt and throw my tray table up and as I'm about to stand up, flight attendant says 'everyone stay calm, it's just a night terror, he is alright.' I continue to watch the scene closely.
>
> "A couple mins later he is unresponsive again and the flight attendant yells "call overhead for a physician on board". I raised my hand to grab her attention. She said to me, "Oh no sweetie put your hand down, we are looking for actual physicians or nurses or some type of medical personnel, we don't have time to talk to you" I tried to inform her that I was a physician but I was continually cut off by condescending remarks.

"Then overhead they paged 'any physician on board please press your button.' I stare at her as I go to press my button. She said 'Oh wow, you're an actual physician?' I reply yes. She said, 'Let me see your credentials. What type of doctor are you? Where do you work? Why were you in Detroit?' (Please remember this man is still in need of help and she is blocking my row from even standing up while bombarding me with questions).

"I respond, 'OBGYN, work in Houston, in Detroit for a wedding, but believe it or not they DO HAVE doctors in Detroit. Now excuse me so I can help the man in need.' Another "seasoned" White male approaches the row and says he is a physician as well. She says to me, 'Thanks for your help but he can help us, and he has his credentials.'" (Mind you, he hasn't shown anything to her. Just showed up and fit the "description of a doctor") I stay seated. Mind blown. Blood boiling. (Man is responding to his questions and is seemingly better now, thank God)

"Then this heifer has the nerve to ask for my input on what to do next about ten mins later. I tell her we need vitals and blood sugar. She comes back to report to me a BP of 80/50 (super low, to my non-medical peeps) and they can't find a glucometer. We continue down that pathway of medical work up, but the point is she needed my help and I continued to help despite the choice words I had saved up for her. The patient and his wife weren't the problem, they needed help and we were midflight.

> "She came and apologized to me several times and offering me SkyMiles. I kindly refused. This is going higher than her. I don't want SkyMiles in exchange for blatant discrimination. Whether this was race, age, gender discrimination, it's not right. She will not get away with this... and I will still get my SkyMiles..."
>
> A close friend of mine had commented under the post to make it "public" so she could share the post from my typically private page. After I played around for ten minutes, I figured out how to change the privacy of the post to public. I never even knew Facebook even had this function! I took my seat, turned my phone to airplane mode, and off to sleep I went in my window seat.

◇◇◇◇◇◇◇◇◇◇◇◇◇◇◇◇◇◇◇◇◇◇◇◇◇◇◇◇◇◇◇◇◇◇◇◇◇◇

Over the past several decades, it has been shown statistically that among doctors, we have essentially closed the gender gap. Headlines in recent years have highlighted the fact that women physicians have finally caught up to male physicians and the disparity is no more. Demographic analysis supports this notion and even supports that women are now surpassing men in matriculation and graduation rates from medical schools across the country. Of all physicians older than 65 years old, males comprised of 82% of them, compared to 56% of physicians between ages 45 to 54 years old, compared to 39% of physicians under the age of 35.

We can be content that we closed this huge gap and celebrate the 53% increase in Black female medical school graduates, but I feel we need to also be concerned for our 39% decrease in Black male medical school graduates since 1986. We can be complacent for how far we have come, or we can continue to work on closing the $80,000 annual pay gap amongst male and female physicians for the exact same jobs. The choice is yours, but I say we still have work to do.

I'm no statistician nor epidemiologist, but to say these numbers I am about to share are ALARMING is an understatement! Fifteen percent of the US population are Black and about eight percent of the US population are Black females. We know this. We are a minority. Let's look at another measure. Five percent of all physicians in this country are Black, and only two percent of physicians are Black females. As if these numbers are not already low enough as is, let's look at the grand scheme of things. Physicians are a minority in this country, making up only a third of a percent of Americans. Do the math. Black physicians make up 0.02 percent of the US population. Black female physicians make up half of that.

I wanted to outline these numbers and walk through the math to really drill in the existing disparities we have in this country. A Black female physician is a rarity compared to the remaining population of physicians. So when we come across one, how do we react? Are we happy for her and praising her achievements? Are we unamused, because it's becoming more increasingly common? Or are we in so much shock that we do not believe it to be true, that this Black woman is actually a doctor?

To be perfectly honest, as a Black female physician and one of the fraction of a percent, I have received all three reactions. I would be lying if I said the varying responses were correlated with race, gender, and age. I have had Black women not believe I was a physician, older White men sing my praises for my accomplishments, and every other kind of combination in between.

If I had a nickel for every time I was "mistaken" for another job other than the physician, I would be able to comfortably retire off my assets by now. I have been mistaken for the medical assistant, janitor, food services, nurse, patient's family member, student, and the list goes on. While all of these are noble professions, why are people assuming my title before I introduce myself? Even better, is AFTER I introduce myself as the doctor, what makes it so confusing that you still do not understand my title as doctor? The simple answer is implicit bias.

Implicit bias is the attitudes and stereotypes that shape our unconscious decisions and understanding. Because one does not see many Black female doctors, as outlined previously, that when a woman introduces herself as such, and has the uniform, badge and title to support it, said person still doesn't "hear" doctor, because of their own implicit bias. Because of the unconscious etiology of implicit bias, it is hard to "blame" a single person for their internal bias that they likely did not know they had. The blame should be directed at the reason why this implicit bias exists in the first place. Our system is broken. Our system is designed to help some, while leave others behind. How do we change that? We need more minority leadership in corporate America. We need more minority leadership in healthcare, specifically. We need more funding of pipeline programs to expose minorities to the "fields" they never dreamed they could tap into. We need for more minorities who hold these sought-after positions to go back into the very communities in which they come from to inspire, educate, and uplift our youth. Most of our youth's dreams are based on things they have seen. The children who aspire to be professional athletes, are likely because they see minority players in the media. More will aspire to be physicians once they see how many of us have achieved it.

Without a family member or role model in medicine to look up to, it's not a reality to them. Think about how many young minorities have started "dreaming to be President of the United States" after they saw President Barack Obama in office for two consecutive terms! Better yet, how many young girls are now dreaming of becoming the next Vice President, following in Madam Vice President, Kamala Harris' footsteps? People need to see that we exist—women physicians, all 0.15% of us. Black physicians, all 0.02% of us. Black women physicians, all 0.01% of us. Our presence is affirmation, confirmation, and motivation to our youth who may strive to one day become what we are.

When I landed in Houston, I took my phone out of airplane mode and checked my messages and Facebook. My post had over 4000 likes and shares! I do not even have 4000 friends! From that moment on, the number of shares and likes climbed exponentially. Reaching over 150,000 likes and over 45,000 shares of my original post (this does not account for the shares and likes of other people's "repost"), people from all over the world were contacting me via email, Facebook, and LinkedIn.

Within just a few days, I had news reporters contacting me, harassing my friends and family and waiting outside of my home and my job. For a private person, this was not a comfortable period of my life. Local Detroit news reporters were knocking on my parents' door in Michigan. My story was on almost every major news station, radio station, talk show, etc. An array of profile pictures from my Facebook account were circling the internet in addition to my work photo on the website. I was overwhelmed by the media attention, but still did not regret it one bit. This story deserved attention and I felt that this was the voice of so many other minority professionals all over this country and the world. The more I saw people sharing similar stories, the more reassured I was that this was the right decision. To be completely transparent, I had days that I wanted to ball up in my bed under the covers, delete the post and act like none of this happened. It was a lot to deal with. How did people find my address? This address was not even listed on any of my documents as I had just purchased the home one year prior. I worked at several different hospitals in residency, so how did they know where I was at what time?

Luckily (or not) I was in the middle of a pretty rigorous and rough rotation that required me to be at work late on many nights, just long enough to avoid the reporters in the parking lot or at my house. I was working 80-hour work weeks and my phone was going off all day and night every single day with texts, emails, messages, etc. Not to mention, I was in the middle of my chief year in residency (last year, when preparing for boards and transitioning out of OBGYN training), and at the peak of interview season. This was NOT what I would call an ideal time to have a post go viral.

Would future job prospects have seen this story? Would they know it was me? Would they ask about it during the interview? Would this impact me getting a job? What if they disagreed with my viral post? What if they felt I was being disruptive? ALL of these questions circled my mind all day, every day. The answer to most of those questions is yes! Many of the media outlets wanted the story immediately so when they had not heard back from me, they wrote that I was avoiding calls. In reality, I was just working. Anyone who has gone through a rigorous residency knows the demanding schedule it requires. I vowed to myself that although I had not planned nor ever imagined this would go viral, I would not let it affect my job. I remember talking with my co-chief Wyntrea who was also a good friend and her being concerned about me and knowing how private I am. She asked if I needed a couple days off. I refused to take any time off. I knew with prayer, perseverance, and time that it would blow over and I could not have asked for a more supportive department and University. I had thousands of Facebook messages and there was no way I could get through all of them as fast as they were coming in. People reached out to me from Nigeria, Trinidad, Ecuador, Venezuela, the list goes on.

Not only was I personally overwhelmed by it all, but I felt extremely guilty. Our department, and program director, and coordinator were receiving calls and emails and letters regarding the situation as well. People were verifying if I was actually a doctor. Some were verifying my age, as they did not believe I could be 28 years old and be a physician (Mind you, I had not told anyone my age, they were getting it from the internet or Facebook etc.). Others were debating that I was not a physician because on the Texas Medical Board website, my license said I was a physician in training. I was exactly that.

To clarify any remaining confusion, I was a physician and I was in training. At the time of this incident, I had successfully completed medical school and had earned my doctorate of medicine and was in the 4th year of my post graduate four-year long OBGYN residency training. Whether it be a nurse or EMT who may have stepped forward, I was just as qualified to assist in this emergency. I had not only received basic life support (BLS) certification, but I also had received Advanced Cardiac Life Support (ACLS) certification. I mean, I am no cardiologist, but being a physician and a graduating chief in a surgical specialty, I was qualified to assist.

Moreover, let's be frank... to all of my healthcare professionals, who is actually excited to answer the infamous "call on board for medical personnel"? Raise your hand higher, we will wait. Exactly. No one. Most of us in the healthcare field actually dread being in this incident. Even if we deal with this day to day, we are over 30,000 feet in the air, in a tight space, with extremely limited resources and little to no help from other trained medical professionals. Who wouldn't be scared? Not to mention the fear of being liable in the event a negative outcome ensues.

We all are taught about the "Good Samaritan Law" that protects us in these types of emergencies, but who wants to test it? We face litigation on the daily with our profession. Who wants to deal with the added stress if we can just stay quiet and let one of the other medical professionals help instead. I'm sharing that to debunk yet another myth. That "Cross was just upset that she did not get to help". No, that is absolutely furthest from the truth. If my morals weren't weighing in as heavily as they do, I would love to sit and watch the rest of my movie and not get caught up in the situation, as I am sure a few other physicians on that plane did that day.

As I watched the wife screaming for help, who in their right mind would just sit and ignore? Even if I wasn't trained to help, I would still run to see how I COULD help. But the mere fact that I would have known if this man needed CPR and I could effectively do that, was enough to make me volunteer without hesitation. Sorry if that made me appear as overzealous and eager. Being a physician comes with an oath, even when we are "off the clock" and a list of medical ethics that we follow. Being a physician goes beyond the confines of the hospital and incorporates treating and caring for your community. This was my goal and will continue to be my goal.

In all of the feedback and responses I received, I would say that over 90% was encouraging and positive. Even though there was no way for me to possibly respond to every email, text, and direct message that I received, I read them all and it was truly warming. I took a leap of faith with sharing my story. Especially during the time I was interviewing and about to start my career. If this was not well received, it could have been career ending. I still continued to see the need for this to be shared and I had to be brave and stand up for what I believed in. As I mentioned previously, me being dismissed as a physician was no new phenomenon. This was my every day since I was a medical student. I knew I was not alone because my colleagues and I have had conversations regarding these hurtful truths.

Do not even get me started on what our Black male physicians have had to endure. The stereotypes have greeted them at the patients' doorstep on many occasions. So we know this is not new. My situation was not unique. The embarrassing truth is that we usually "brush them off" and eventually become desensitized to them. I could have easily done that with this situation. My reasoning for not doing so was two-fold. First, this was a major safety concern and could potentially impact future passengers and needed to be addressed on a higher level. Secondly, I was tired of quietly ignoring these commonly occurring situations.

If one only knew the strides that my colleagues and I had to make to get to where we stand today; the hard work, sleepless nights, tears, and sacrifices that not only we had to make, but our friends and family had to make to accommodate our "lifelong dream", then you would understand the infuriation. To repetitively have someone dismiss you and your hard-earned credentials within seconds isn't exactly a warm feeling. The other issue I saw was that although amongst us minorities, we know this to be true, but what does everyone else know? So many friends and colleagues were in disbelief that this actually happens daily. We needed our story told—publicly—and this served as a platform to do just that. So I did.

The amount of support I received from women and men of all ethnic backgrounds had me in tears. People who never met me, who supported me, who shared my story, who shared our hashtag, #whatadoctorlookslike, were coming together to have this uncomfortable national conversation. This became a movement in which people posted pictures of themselves or friends with the tag #whatadoctorlookslike to share that despite the bias and stereotypes, doctors come in all genders, ethnic backgrounds, and age. I was prevented from helping because I did not fit the "mold" of what the flight attendant thought a doctor looked like: a young Black woman from Detroit, in a hoodie and leggings.

Several articles were published with women coming forward sharing their stories of when their help was "denied" due to implicit bias. This was affirmation. Not that I needed further affirmation, because I lived this truth my whole life. But our broken society needed affirmation from other sources than the "young Black girl who is trying to get on the Today Show". People's eyes began to open and the problem became bigger than me and people started truly understanding the core of the discussion.

As previously mentioned, the majority of feedback was supportive and heartwarming, but it came with negative feedback as well. I read very hateful and hurtful comments on the thread as well as several emails. From racial slurs to people thinking I made the entire story up. I guess I did not have anything better to do with my time. Ha! I even had a couple people go on different physician rating websites to give a negative review, despite not having ever met me nor been my patient. I saw comments of people saying that I did this looking for media attention. Right. Which is why I turned down every TV opportunity offered (and there were several), did minimal phone interviews only to get "my story out".

If I was looking for the limelight, I definitely could have capitalized on this situation to go on every news channel and be flown out to meet various people around the country. My focus was not on me and "how I felt". My focus was on the greater message of implicit bias and its effects in the workplace. My goal was to tell my story which wasn't only my story, but so many hundreds of thousands of people's stories. When I realized how many people this situation resonated with, I was reassured that this needed to be said and I had done the right thing by not being quiet.

So I took the negativity in stride and stuck to my overarching goals: Keep the conversation going, educate people on implicit bias, encourage all of us to explore are inner biases and work to not let them affect our daily decisions. I also wanted to reach more youth by fostering mentorship so we have more diversity in the medical field. With more diversity, there will be no single prototype of #whatadoctorlookslike, but the profile will be such a wide array of ages, gender, ethnicity, background, and sexuality.

Because the airlines insisted that the flight attendant was following an outdated policy, I sat down with the executives of the company to discuss this policy that was inconsistently enforced. During several phone conversations and meetings at the airline's headquarters in Atlanta, Georgia, we discussed the flaws in this outdated policy that was not routinely or equally enforced. I brought with me to the meeting, Dr. Wayne J. Riley, the former president of my medical school, past president of the American College of Physicians, and a mentor of mine. He was well-versed on flight emergencies as evidenced by a routine lecture he gave during our capstone course before graduating from Meharry.

We finally were able to make change. As of December 1st, 2016, the airlines implemented a new policy that did not require medical professionals to produce credentials prior to assisting in an emergency. They would be able to state their credentials and help with initial assessment. Later after the passenger is stabilized, or needing a higher level of care, they will further verify credentials. Also on this date, the airline implemented new cultural sensitivity and bias training for all employees. Some people argued this was not enough and they needed to do more, but honestly, I was content that this negative situation was able to change a longstanding policy of one of the biggest companies in the world.

Speaking up and standing your ground is important. Of course, we must choose our battles wisely, but you never know the impact you have on others unless you speak up. Your voice is more powerful than you think. I did not think that by sharing my story on social media, it would spread like wildfire reaching major media outlets and eventually producing meaningful change.

Now...

More than four years have passed. Being remote from the situation is always a good time for reflection. Do I feel this made a difference? Absolutely. This incident sparked a post which sparked a movement which opened an important conversation. There have been so many articles and books published regarding this topic, some indirectly or directly referencing my story. I feel that by me sharing this with the world, I was able to help open up this topic of discussion and bring awareness to something that we had all been dealing with for decades.

Do I regret my post? Definitely not. I prayed about it then, and pray about it now and I know that God intended for me to help shape people's views and awareness of this matter.

I have been asked several times do I dress more "professional" or "business casual" on a plane as a result of this situation. The simple answer is no. I still wear the very things I wore back in October 2016. With that being said, I do want to highlight the importance of looking well kempt and presentable, not only as a lady, but as a professional. Although I wore a sweatshirt that day, I wasn't "unkempt" or unprofessional and I would still wear the exact same thing if traveling between a cold and hot climate. Let's be honest, I get mistaken as the janitor when I have on a suit, white coat, and badge, so is it really the attire that is "confusing people"? I'll let you, dear reader, be the judge of that.

Did I sue the airlines and win a ton of money or fly free for the rest of my life? No. I did not file a lawsuit against the airline, because with the implementation of new policy and programs, I was content with the resolution. I wish I flew free for life. I still purchase my plane tickets like everyone else. My goal was not for a financial gain or a "come up". My goal was to share my story in hopes of implementing change.

Although I initially turned down more than twenty requests to be on various shows discussing this incident, it doesn't mean that I haven't been able to reap opportunities from the situation. I have had several requests to speak to students or in forums regarding the pathway to become a doctor. This is priceless. Not only have I always had a passion for mentorship, but it's comforting to know we are finally moving past what happened on Flight DL945 and onto the bigger issue. Let's reach out to the community and our youth to help breed young doctors or other healthcare professionals.

In my home church, Higher Dimension in Houston, I was blessed to have a pastor and first lady who supported me through that difficult and overwhelming point in my life. The motto of our church is, "Love God, love people, and reach the community". This is the best summary of exactly what I am striving to do.

Affirmation to recite*: I belong here. I am qualified.*

Question*: Have you ever had your credentials questioned? How did that make you feel? Did it make you feel like you didn't belong? How did you handle that situation?*

Part V

The Butterfly (Attending)

CHAPTER 16

Sitting on the Other Side of the Table

"God has a purpose for your pain, a reason for your struggles, and a reward for your faithfulness. Don't give up."

-Eric Thomas

"Hello, it's Dr. Cross with OBGYN, how can I help you?" I answered my work phone. It had been a long busy day at work. Two days out of the week I worked as an OBGYN hospitalist taking all the consultations for the entire hospital. The phone had been ringing non-stop all day and my shift was coming to a close in just 30 minutes.

"Hey Dr. Cross, we have a patient down in the emergency room who is having a miscarriage and bleeding pretty heavily. She is in Trauma Bay #3. Can you please come down to assist us?" the ER doctor requested.

"Sure thing, I will be right there. Please make sure she has two large bore IVs in place and order a CBC and Type and Screen STAT!" I hurry off the phone to get to the ER and assist with this emergent consult. By the time we stabilized the patient and the bleeding came to a stop, it was an hour past the end of my shift. I gave my report to the night shift doctor and headed out to the parking lot.

Driving home in rush hour traffic was always a task in Houston, but after living here for several years, you get used to the traffic and make sure you have good music or an audiobook for the ride. I was riding northbound on the 288 freeway. As you begin to approach the center of the city, the freeway splits and I head toward the Midtown exit where I lived at the time.

BOOM!

My car spun around full circle faster than I could realize what had just happened. A car from the other side of the split decided last minute to come to my lane and hit the gas full speed head on into the passenger side of my car. My tire was blown out and I lost complete control of the right side of my car which threw me into the next lane. Being that it was a busy freeway, I could have easily been hit by multiple cars. I know "Jesus take the wheel" is a phrase, but that was exactly what happened there.

By the grace of God, I was able to maneuver my car in a way to stop my car from flying across any more lanes. Both cars came to a complete stop. My entire body was shaking uncontrollably. I was terrified. I looked down at my arms and legs. Not one single scratch on me. After a few seconds flew by, I jumped into action. I pressed my SOS button in the car to notify police and send help.

I hopped out my car and ran over to the brand new Chrysler 300 that had just hit my three-month-old BMW grand coupe. There was a young nervous, frantic 20-year-old girl behind the wheel. She rolled her window down and apologized profusely to me.

"I am so sorry, I was trying to change to a different lane so I could exit and I did not see you! I am so sorry, please..." I cut her off.

"Are you ok? Can you get out of the car, please. Do you have any injuries? The paramedics are on the way, but I am a doctor and I can help you until they arrive." I reassured her. She started crying.

"Oh my God, I am so sorry. I don't know how this happened. I am ok. I am not injured, are you? You're being so nice to me!" she replied.

"No, I am not hurt either. It's a blessing that we are both ok." I responded. We then proceeded to exchange information. The police arrived at the scene, issued her a ticket for the accident and driving without a license apparently. Paramedics arrived to the scene, examined and interviewed us both. I declined all medical care. I was fine. I'll probably have some soreness tomorrow so I'll take a couple ibuprofens before bed and I'll be alright. Four hours later, my car was finally towed to a collision shop and I was back in my apartment.

That's when it all hit. I literally had this brand new car for three months and within the blink of an eye, an uninsured driver without a license, T-boned me and totaled it. What a day. I cried myself to sleep that night.

The next morning I woke up, and as expected, I was sore all over. The ibuprofen sure didn't feel like it had done anything. I went to grab my glasses and that's when I realized my hands felt funny. I had decreased sensation and a tingling feeling that was more pronounced on my left side. I replayed the accident in my head over and over again trying to figure out the etiology for my symptoms. Go figure. I am a surgeon and I need my hands. This was the only reason I took myself to the nearest emergency room to get imaging done.

This accident came completely out the blue flying full speed. I never thought that I would ever be T-boned on the freeway. To this day when I tell people that, they always have to circle back and make sure I said that correctly. Yep. T-boned on the freeway when all traffic should be going the same direction. My previous car, I had for 12 years and I rode that thing until the wheels fell off... literally. Then three months with my "new baby" and it was totaled out with over $50,000 worth of damage. But in the end, this accident saved my life; a true blessing in disguise.

The imaging and doctors' visits that were initiated as a result of the car accident ended up leading to an incidental finding of a 15-cm solid tumor growing inside my abdomen. I always knew I was only human and things could happen to me, but I always felt some element of being invincible. I think many healthcare providers can relate. To go from always being the caregiver and the doctor and the problem solver, to now being the vulnerable patient, scared and in shock, was an eye opener for me. Ignorance is truly bliss. Knowing too much can be a blessing and a curse. Navigating the medical process as a medical professional, your breadth of knowledge can literally drive you crazy. You must learn to turn off the provider hat, and just be patient, and be a patient.

After multiple tests, it still was not clear what the mass was. *Was it cancer? If so, had it spread? Where was this tumor coming from? How long had it been there?* The best answer my doctor could conjure up was, "I do not know if it is cancer, it does not exactly look like cancer, but it looks concerning and is very large, so it must come out. It appears to be attached to either your adrenal gland, kidney, spleen, or pancreas. We do not see anything else concerning for spread elsewhere but this needs to come out sooner than later. I wouldn't wait."

To non-medical people this may be interpreted as, "We are not sure what it is, but probably not cancer. Let's take it out and we will have more answers."

To me as a medical provider it was interpreted as, "This thing looks like cancer but I do not want to scare you right now until we know for sure. If it's coming from your kidney, you'll lose it, and possibly go on dialysis. If it's coming from your pancreas, you'll be dead in 6 months because pancreatic cancer has one of the worse prognoses. If it is coming from your spleen or adrenal, that is best case scenario, but you still need a major surgery and will be out from work for several weeks."

I mean on top of being a doctor, I may be a little neurotic. Either way, the second interpretation was definitely how my brain took the news.

I prayed. My family prayed. My few friends I had opened up to about it prayed. Four days after my 30th birthday, I underwent a six-hour surgery to remove the tumor. My left adrenal gland and part of my left kidney were removed during the surgery in order to get the entire tumor out. My pancreas and spleen were able to be carefully peeled from the tumor and it had not invaded those organs. I give God all the glory.

Before I made the decision to completely give it all to God, I had a great deal of worry in my heart. I was so used to being the one in the operating room holding the knife, that I did not know how things would go as me being under the knife. I wanted to see what they were doing, make sure they didn't cut anything that didn't need to be cut, make sure they kept my blood loss to a minimum, and also, I wanted to make sure they sewed up my incision and made it look pretty! Summer was only a couple months away! But in actuality, this worry was good even if I only felt for a few moments.

I do really well in empathizing with my patients before and after surgery, but this would make me empathize on a different level. I had minor procedures done in the past, but never one this big, and never with this much element of the unknown. This is how so many of my patients felt—having surgery to have fibroids removed and knowing that they may lose their entire uterus and ability to bear children while they are asleep if any unexpected bleeding occurred, or having surgery to remove a complex cyst that appeared to be benign but might end up being cancer and needing their uterus, both ovaries and lymph nodes removed. This made me love my patients even more than I already did and that is saying a lot! The level of trust I had to have in my urologist to perform such a major surgery on a control freak is off the charts.

So when my patients are choosing me as their obstetrician or their surgeon or gynecologist, they are trusting me with their life, their health, and even their child's life when I am caring for their pregnancy. Wearing the shoes of my patients for some time allowed me to peek into the vulnerability, the fear, the confusion, and frustration they may feel at times. This has contributed greatly in molding and defining me as the physician I am today.

This accident was a blessing in disguise. I can't lie...

I was upset. An uninsured driver without a license, Lord? Seriously? My brand new coupe completely totaled?

I was afraid. Am I dying? Will I need chemotherapy and radiation? Will I still be able to have kids? Will I be around for next Christmas?

I was hurt. Going through my recovery process many people close to me who I thought would be there, were absent. Are they avoiding me because they think I am dying? Why won't they come visit me? Did they forget about me?

The biggest thing was that I was alive, I was healthy, and on my way to strengthening my spiritual, physical, emotional, and psychological health.

Think about your circle of friends or family. It may be a large circle or a small circle. You may all be from the same hometown or from all over. Your circle may consist of only one gender or ethnicity or have a mixture. Your circle is who you go to in a time of need; your core group of people. Now think about who in your circle most would classify as "the strong friend". You know, the friend who is always there for everyone else, but seemingly always strong. The friend who never seems to have any problems that he or she may seek counsel about. The friend who you never see cry. If you cannot think of who it is, think harder. Every circle has at least one.

It is possible that if you are having difficulty identifying said person, then quite possibly, it may be you. Regardless of your chill, zen, have-it-all-together exterior, the truth is that you're human. You have the same issues as your friends, you just carry it differently, possibly by hiding it. You're not exempt from the ups and downs and emotional rollercoasters of bullshit that plagues everyone else. You just simply cover it up better than most. That's all.

I won't go too hard on you, because honestly, I am that friend too. I am the strong one, who never needs help, seemingly has it all together, navigates life's emotional rollercoasters with a smile. Yep, that's me. The strong friend is the one everyone goes to for advice, resources, prayer, or just simply a pep talk. It's an honorable hat to wear amongst your circle of friends, so you should be proud. The downfall is that the "strong friend" can be stubborn when it comes to asking for and accepting help from others.

It's actually pretty hypocritical when you think about it. You want everyone to trust you and open up to you, but in reality, you're faking the funk like all is well. It isn't that you try to come off as such, but your wall isn't exactly let down to allow your most trusted friends and family see deeper into your emotions like you expect of them. I know this role all too well, and have learned to be vulnerable with those whom I love and trust.

The strong friend doesn't boast about his or her strength. It is an innate personality trait that can be hard to overcome. Just because everyone thinks you have it all together certainly does not mean that you do. It is merely how others perceive you without you shouting to the world that you're strong and happy and have a perfect life. I have learned that because the strong friend is always perceived as having life figured out, no one in your circle is ever expecting you to be the one seeking counsel. Since you carry yourself in such a way that everyone cannot always tell that something is wrong or you need something, you have to pretty much come out and ask for it. This is something the strong friend does not routinely do. We would rather just keep it to ourselves and go about our day. No harm done, right? Wrong.

When the strong friend needs help, wants company, or a shoulder to cry on, but does not know how to directly express that, the default is to keep quiet. The problem weighs in because although the strong friend is keeping to himself, he is lowkey resenting others for not extending a helping hand, as said friend has done for others for the past five, ten, fifteen years. That's not fair to your circle. Exchange your resentment for understanding.

It took me some time to realize that this was me through and through. As I navigated my silent obstacles and shortcomings and insecurities quietly, I continued to hear from others how perfect my life appeared. I never boasted a perfect life. Hell my life wasn't perfect. I then began to realize that often times, when others don't see you sweat, they cannot appreciate the challenges you have overcome to get where you are. Although it was frustrating that my many obstacles were glossed over, I soon began to embrace the fact that I carried myself in such a way. It actually served as a confidence booster in many ways. Until it bit me in the ass one day...

As I mentioned, when I dealt with a tough season in my life, with seemingly problem after problem, I faced a period of time where I felt very alone. From having to back out of a contract on a new house that was infiltrated with damage from a catastrophic hurricane that hit Houston, to finding a place to live within 48 hours, to totaling my brand new sports car, to being diagnosed with a huge tumor with an unknown prognosis, amongst other things, within a three-month span, I was drowning.

Apparently, my head was still above water, just enough to let my circle know I was alive, but beneath the surface, I was drowning. I called on friends and family to share my experiences but to my surprise, I still felt very alone. I remember after my crazy car accident, being shook and scared. Somehow, I still managed to effortlessly speak with a calm voice. I called one of my closest friends and explained what had happened and that I needed a ride. She responded that she would come "after she is done cooking dinner". I remember being pissed, but more importantly hurt. This was a friend who I would have dropped everything to come assist during a time in need, especially if I knew she did not have any family in town. Once we were able to sit down and discuss the issue (which was several weeks later), she said something that I knew was true. She was apologetic, and explained that she did not realize the gravity of the situation because of how calm I sounded on the phone. Yes I was pissed, resulting in the several week-long hiatus I took, but I knew that was no exaggeration and I probably did not sound panicky. Strong friend syndrome at its best.

Another example was when I was in the hospital after my surgery for the tumor. I had people reach out and ask me if I needed anything. That is probably one of the most cringeworthy questions to ask someone during a time of need. I am guilty of it too. Sometimes it is just best, to be there, to be present, regardless if they aren't requesting anything specific. During that time, I appreciated the calls and prayers and people stopping by to see me. Yes I looked like crap and was high off drugs the first day or two in the hospital, but presence was truly the best present for me. When some of the closest people to me didn't show up (literally and figuratively), it felt like a slap in the face. Again, that strong friend syndrome struck again.

I seemed like I was good, did not need anything, and did not ask for anything. On the inside, I was scared, depressed, in pain, and I felt empty. Empty because many of the people I have showed up for or would show up for, did not show up for me. I began to resent people. Family. Friends. Everyone. This only made me feel worse inside and created a self-pity that I hate thinking about to this day. I was hurt that my people were not there for me in the way I needed them to be. In reality, they did not know how to be there for me, because I was the strong friend. I hadn't needed them to be there for me before and I sure as hell did not know how to communicate when I did.

I wasn't ok, and that's alright. It was a humbling experience. One day, I was riding around in my sports car, visiting friends and family, working, and getting back in shape. Just a couple months later, I was laying in a hospital bed, needing help to wipe my butt, tie my shoes, and shower, all while wondering how close I was to death. It was a horrible feeling and although no one could take that nasty feeling away, presence is comforting during those times. Being asked 1000 times what kind of tumor it was and if it was cancerous and what am I going to do was not comforting at all. I did not have any answers for weeks. Those weeks felt like years and the more people that asked me about it, the more anxious I grew. Again, no malicious intent with asking, but since I did not know how to communicate to people "shut the hell up" in a nice way, I just gritted my teeth and answered each time with a smile.

We all are different, but for me, the hardest part of this process was the unknown. We had so many unknowns going into surgery. We did not know if it was going to be spread throughout my abdomen, or if it was coming from my kidney or pancreas or adrenal gland or if it was going to be resectable and how many complications would occur in trying to remove it. The doctor in me would spend hours every single night looking up papers on various types of tumors and the prognosis. I became obsessed with it. I stared at statistics for every potential tumor in the abdomen. I looked up all the potential treatments depending on what it would be. I drove myself insane, but I hated not knowing. We did MRIs, CT scans, ultrasounds and lab work, and nothing was definitive. I had to get to a point of turning it over to God because there was nothing I could do to control the situation any more.

After surgery, we had more answers, but not a ton. We knew it was coming from the adrenal gland and not from the spleen, kidney, pancreas. We knew it was solid and no contents appeared spilled into my abdomen. It appeared that he had removed the entire tumor and that was great news. We did not know if it was cancerous or not. We did not know how we were going to treat it if it was. We did not know if I would need chemotherapy or radiation or a combination of both. We did not know if it was going to come back and if it was, we did not know when. I wanted more answers.

Initially, the pathology was supposed to be back in three days. Those three days turned into weeks. We came to find out that this tumor had never been seen before by the top pathologists in the world, including the doctors at MD Anderson Cancer Center—one of the best in the world. What took so long was that my tumor was being passed around to various facilities trying to figure out what this thing was. It was so rare, it was not in the textbooks and there was no specified regimen on how to treat it. My final pathology came back as "unknown malignant potential".

In layman's terms, it was not normal enough to call benign, but not atypical enough to call it cancerous. In gynecology, we call these "borderline" tumors. This answer was not good enough for the doctor in me. Being rare and unique is usually a great characteristic, but in the medical world, no one wants to be rare. So essentially, we had to devise a surveillance plan. It consisted of routine imaging tests for the next five years. These tumors typically recur in the first five years so once we are out of that range, we have low suspicion for it coming back. There was nothing I could do to prevent it. It placed me in "limbo" for five years.

My non-medical family and friends would cheer me up, saying things like, "Well at least you don't have cancer and this is all over". Although it was supposed to be a comforting word, it was not comforting to me. *How did they know it was not cancer, if the top doctors in the world did not know what the hell it was?* People hear what they want to hear and try to hang on to the silver lining to get through tough times. The realist in me would get so frustrated with that comment. I did not want to be pessimistic, but I knew that I was going to be the one dealing with the anxiety for the next five years.

To everyone else, it was over. Tamika was back to work in no time and back to her regular routine with ease. Crisis averted. What my circle did not know was the extreme anxiety attacks I developed every time I went into the MRI machine and laid there for hours, meditating and calming myself down. Or the anxiety I developed when I sat in the doctor's office waiting for the results every 6 months. I had never dealt with anxiety prior to then so this was all new for me. There I was, Dr. Cross, with a newly developed fear of doctors. Go figure. It's almost laughable at this point, but it sure as hell was not funny at that time.

Although the experience was a difficult one for me to navigate, I still think it helped me empathize with my patients even more than I previously did. Unknown territory is always scary, so it's essential to have a great team of friends, family, and healthcare professionals by your side. My doctor was great. He explained everything to me in detail, outlined our management plan, and talked me "off a cliff" every time I had my mini panic attacks in his office. He would pause, stare at me, smile and then offer a comforting word or two. This always brought me back to the ground and made me feel better. I could not have chosen a better team to care for me.

As for my circle, it took me one to two years and several therapy sessions to be able to express myself to them. I found that journaling helped as well. I also found that it is helpful to share your testimony with others when you're ready. You never know whose life you may be saving by sharing your story. Some people just want to know they are not alone.

To my fellow "strong friends", it is ok to be vulnerable sometimes and let your hair down. We all need somebody. If you are not usually the one in need, it may be a new phenomenon for your friends helping you navigate difficult times, so be patient with them. Be open and direct with your needs. If you want them to sit and watch TV with you and be quiet, say that. Always remember that presence can sometimes be the best present. Embrace your circle. They love you and appreciate you and want to be there for you. There may be some people who you realize are only there for the high times and disappear during the low times. It's ok. They may have already served their purpose in your life in a different season. Let them exit your life quietly, and you focus your time and energy on those who celebrate you during both the good and bad.

Affirmation to recite: *I will be the best version of myself and I will give others grace as they navigate being the best version of themselves as well.*

Question: *When have you faced a difficult season in your life and were seemingly all alone? Who did you reach out to? How did you navigate that tough season? Do you handle situations differently now as a result?*

CHAPTER 17

Primum Non Nocere

"Differences of race, nationality or religion should not be used to deny any human being citizenship rights or privileges."

—Rosa Parks

May 18, 2013 was a day I will never forget. It was hot, humid, the sun was beating down causing me to sweat within five minutes outside. Most importantly, it was the day I graduated from medical school. The heavy graduation garb we were suited in as we were handed our doctoral degree added to the beads of sweat I felt on every single part of my body, but I wore it with pride. I watched classmates who were in a rush to take off the hot robe due to the extreme temperatures outside. I was sweating, and my freshly flat-ironed hair was starting to curl up and expand rapidly under my hat, but you couldn't pay me to take that robe off in that moment.

My medical school, Meharry, in the heart of Nashville, Tennessee, traditionally had our commencement at the infamous Grand Ole Opry House. It was a beautiful ceremony with my classmates who had now become like extended family. Just after we were hooded and back in our respective seats, we were asked to stand for the citing of the Hippocratic Oath. This oath has been historically cited by new physicians for hundreds of years and was originally written in Latin. There have been many different versions and revisions made over the years.

One of the major components included in the oath is: "I will remember that there is an art to medicine as well as science and that warmth, sympathy, and understanding may outweigh the surgeon's knife or the chemist's drug." This speaks to the notion that although we study the medicine and science, we are also human and treating other humans. It is important to encompass empathy in dealing with patients and their health.

Personally, I frequently picture myself in the patients' shoes or treat them as if they were a close family member of mine. *How would I explain this medical condition to my mother? How would I break the unfortunate news to my aunt? How would I offer sympathy through a difficult situation to my grandma?* Doing this helps me personalize the situation and aids me in honoring the Hippocratic Oath. As a surgeon who frequently deals with surgical emergencies and major surgeries, it is easy to become desensitized as means of "survival". We have to be strong, direct, and think with our mind and not our heart in many difficult situations. But the delivery is just as important.

I have learned to sit down at a patient's bedside, with uncrossed arms when discussing important matters. Body language is extremely important and can have a huge impact on the patient and their family members. If a spouse or parent is not present in the hospital during your discussion, you pick up the phone and dial them in. Make them a part of the conversation (only if the patient consents to it of course). These gestures that seem small and subtle to us, make a world of a difference to our patients.

The Hippocratic Oath also states: "If it is given me to save a life, all thanks. But it may also be within my power to take a life; this awesome responsibility must be faced with great humbleness and awareness of my own frailty. Above all, I must not play God." This highlights the importance of our job as physicians. We have the power to save lives or in unfortunate situations, take lives. Although we aren't acting as God, it is through our hands that He has called us to treat patients. With thoughtlessness and carelessness, our mistakes can cost someone their life. This is not in the oath to scare physicians, but to merely remind them of the power their position holds. Because of this power, we must be sure not to abuse it and make sure that we are operating with sane, sound, and unbiased minds.

Because we are human, we will experience the ups and downs that life brings. Oftentimes, we have to put ourselves and our families on the back burner to tend to the patients that need us. A common principle taught in medical school ethics is "primum non nocere" which translates to "first do no harm". This is a short yet very powerful phrase. I keep this in mind for personal practice as well as my team. When we are not able to function at our best, we are doing a disservice to the patients and their loved ones.

In the medical field, it is common for us to begin to feel that we can work through tough emotional, physical, and psychological periods in our life. We were built tough and have overcome so much that we feel that we can push forward. I am guilty of feeling that way in the past as well. Through experience and wisdom, I have learned that when we come to work and aren't functioning at our best, our patients suffer. If you are going through a difficult divorce with your spouse, you received a terrible diagnosis, you lost a close family member or friend, or whatever the case may be, sometimes we are so affected that we cannot safely work and put patient's lives in our hands. Taking time off should not be seen as a weakness, but a strength in these difficult situations.

Working in the medical field is quite often selfless. Most of us go into the medical field because we enjoy tapping into our altruistic spirits to help others. In school, you learn the science, the medicine, and the clinical scenarios you may face. We don't learn much about the sacrifices you must make being a healthcare worker. This job carries such a heavy responsibility, that it is not for the faint of heart. Even when we are not "on the clock", if someone falls ill and we have the capacity to render aid, we have an ethical obligation to assist. It may sound like an easy task, but it's a heavy responsibility to bear. Furthermore, you must know when your burden is more than you can tolerate. If you are going through a rough patch personally, it is ok to take the time you need to recover. Without you being fully functional, you are putting many lives in danger. I cannot stress the importance of self-care when you work in a service-oriented industry. Take the time off when you need it and don't let anybody make you feel bad for it.

I have always been the person who is such a hardworker that I never want to take time off. Sometimes I have to be forced to take time off, because without it, I will keep going. When I faced my medical challenges, I truly believe it was God's way of telling me I needed a break and needed to sit down. The subtle hints and signs were ignored by me until I reached a roadblock so large that I could not ignore it. I remember at work there were a few administrative staff that didn't know much about me, but always had an opinion. Being that I was social and talked to so many people in the department, even at other locations, things always got back to me, even if I didn't want them to.

I remember two workers specifically, Lynn and Eva. Although they were nurse managers and not my boss, they were responsible for schedules and as such and were upset anytime a doctor took off. They had to then reschedule patients and move them around and this required additional work and it simply "was not fair" to them. They bashed me and discussed me every chance they could when I took off work. I had several weeks of saved up sick and vacation time that was mine to take so I didn't understand why I was being bullied into feeling bad for taking it. You truly never know what someone is going through, and sometimes it's best to keep quiet if you don't know. Additionally, when it's not your business, it is best to keep quiet as well.

As much as they bashed me and labeled me "lazy" and would send a series of emails and calls to bully me into working shifts instead of taking off, one would think they would take the time to understand why I was taking off. In a two-year span, I underwent five surgical procedures. With all things considered, the minimal time I took off was negligible. I wasn't vacationing around Europe, but quite frankly, even if I was, that's no one's business. We have sick time and vacation time for a reason, so we really have to get out of the mindset of making people feel guilty who take it or bullying them into coming back to work earlier than their doctor has recommended.

One of the surgeries I had during that series of five was an anterior cruciate ligament (ACL) reconstruction for a completely ruptured ACL along with a fracture to my tibia. When I tell y'all those were the worst two years of my life, I am not exaggerating! That surgery was more of an inconvenience than anything. The rehabilitation of learning how to walk again was humbling. I was determined to come back after a couple weeks, even on crutches, with a full leg brace on, but of course I couldn't deliver babies like that nor operate. My surgeon was extremely nervous about me going back to work because he said one slip on fluids or blood or anything would have me back at square one, requiring surgery and another new ACL.

After convincing him that I would be confined to the office and not working in the hospital, he was ok with me returning to work with those restrictions and taking frequent breaks to sit down and rest my leg. Can you believe that one of the administrative physicians at my job called me and asked me to come back to the hospital? Her justification was that I could use a scooter like some other doctors used after an ankle or Achilles tendon surgery. I was confused because my surgery was on my knee and I could not bend my knee 90 degrees to ride the damn scooter she was referring to and wasn't going to risk tearing something up by going to the hospital before I could walk. Not to mention, it places patients at risk as well. I cannot hustle to an emergent surgery or delivery of a baby on crutches. For the majority of the shifts I worked, I was the only OBGYN in the hospital and there would be no one else to help out on those emergencies. That wasn't safe and I was appalled that I was being asked to do that.

My job as a physician is to first do no harm and that would be a complete violation of that. Tamika a few years prior would have allowed the peer pressure to convince her to do something that she felt was unsafe. But at that time, I stood my ground and told her no. So often, the vibe at work is shame people for taking off, but in actuality the point of it is for us to reset and heal properly when we are ill or have medical issues. We really need to change this across every industry. No one should feel scared or guilty for taking time off work. If you're ill, take off. If you need a personal day, take off. If we don't take care of ourselves, how can we be the best version of ourselves and provide the best care for our patients? In the healthcare sector, a tired, burnt out, or ill physician is dangerous. There are several studies that look at malpractice cases and outcomes when physicians are burned out or tired, which is why so many laws and policies have been put in place to protect them and protect our patients.

Now that leads me to another component of the oath that states: "I will remember that I remain a member of society, with special obligations to all my fellow human beings, those sound of mind and body as well as the infirm." These special obligations to all fellow human beings speak to the responsibility mentioned above. This is the part of the oath that most non-medical folks love to bring to our attention. If someone is choking when I am out at a restaurant, family members or friends love volunteering my assistance, "Tamika, you're a doctor, go help them!" I am sure my medical colleagues can relate to this awkward volunteering that happens quite frequently in public.

The 2020 COVID-19 pandemic was another example of the selfless and unrelenting assistance that medical professionals offered, with significant sacrifices on the line. Within weeks, the world was turned upside down as the pandemic continued to spread from country to country. With several months of warnings, our country was ill prepared with inadequate personal protective equipment, testing swabs and the labs to run the tests in a timely manner. This undoubtedly will make the history books as unprecedented times. A country that we all consider rich in resources, now with limited availability of resources to combat the highly infectious and deadly respiratory virus.

Due to this virus being thought to be spread by small droplets, we had to implement strict measures to attempt to slow the transmission rate. People were instructed to practice social distancing and avoiding contact with people from other households. When in public, people were ordered to remain more than six feet from one another and to wear masks all the time. The world literally shut down. Businesses, schools, and churches were closed. Many people lost their jobs and had no source of income except minimal governmental assistance. Everyone was ordered to stay in their house except for necessities like food and doctor's visits. You can imagine that if doctor's visits and hospitals were an exception, all the healthcare workers continued business as usual. We had to continue to go to work and render aid to those in need, despite increased work hours and significant salary reductions. For me in particular, as an OBGYN, babies were still being born and emergency surgeries still needed to be performed, so for us, we kept working. The difference now being that this deadly and highly infectious virus was floating around from person to person and the most vulnerable and sick people went to the hospital or doctor's office. We screened patients with a couple of questions and a temperature check, trusting that all patients were telling the truth. Go figure.

Due to our country's lack of preparedness, we did not have enough personal protective equipment even for healthcare workers. We ran out of N95 respirator masks, which was recommended to filter out the tiny droplets or aerosols. Then we were told by the governmental agencies that we could just wear surgical masks. When those were running low, we were told we could wear bandanas as makeshift masks in efforts to reduce droplet transmission. Pause. Yes, bandanas. The cloth items that are sold at the beauty supply stores. The cloth items people put on their head at night. These would now suffice as adequate protection per the governmental agencies.

Healthcare workers continued going to work, knowing that they may possibly be exposed to the deadly virus without properly protecting themselves. We continued to care for the patients in need, not knowing what we were carrying home on our clothes or on our bodies and transmitting to our loved ones. We continued to go to work and comfort patients when in reality, we were not comforted ourselves. Pregnant healthcare workers continued working in these dangerous environments because they knew if they stopped going to work, their job may be at risk and they needed the money for their unborn child. Healthcare workers with chronic medical conditions like asthma, diabetes, lung disease, immunosuppression, and cancer continued working for the same reason. Healthcare workers who tested positive for the disease were instructed to slap a mask on and practice rigorous handwashing while still coming to work. Then as more data unfolded about the virus, it was discovered that many people could be asymptomatic carriers; meaning they felt fine, looked fine, and had no symptoms of the disease, yet were passing the disease to everyone they came in contact with.

Work became even scarier. Every person you came in contact with could have this deadly disease, but now we were in close quarters with them, touching things they were touching, praying that the mask they had on their face was adequate at preventing transmission, even though science told us it was not. This was a difficult time for healthcare workers. We had a shortage of workers, because many were simply not willing to risk their lives or the lives of their loved ones and they quit their jobs. Who can blame them? Then all while enduring these crazy times, healthcare workers face the negative comments from non-essential workers.

"You signed up for this, not me. Deal with it."

"You get paid the big bucks to deal with these types of things. Stop complaining."

"At least you get to go to work every day. I have to sit in the house and teach my bad ass kids all day. We are bored!"

Those are a few of the types of comments that were being taunted with as healthcare workers. Unappreciative, inconsiderate comments from people who were tucked away safely in their homes with their loved ones at arms' length. While many hurtful and negative comments were heard, there was a load of positive and appreciative comments from people as well. Local companies were paying for meals for hospital workers or giving discounts at their establishments to honor healthcare workers. Local residents near hospitals cheered and held up signs thanking healthcare workers. It was a warm feeling many days. Regardless if the feedback was positive or negative that day, we had to continue doing our job. That is the type of sacrifice healthcare workers make every single day.

I do not recommend going into the healthcare field if you are not passionate about it. With the amount of sacrifices you and your family have to make on a daily basis, it truly is not worth it if the passion is not in it. For me, my passion drives me to go back day in and day out and have no regrets. Without the dedication to this dream, I would have quit ages ago. Make sure your fire is being fueled by the right reasons.

This COVID-19 pandemic unveiled many of the ugly disparities that exist in healthcare. Black people were dying at a rate more than other ethnicities. My hometown, Detroit, Michigan, remained in the top 10 cities in the country that was hit the hardest throughout the entire pandemic. Statistically, Detroit is literally the Blackest city in America with a population that is more than 80% Black. So it is no surprise to many of us that we were hit the hardest despite not being as large of a metropolis as New York City that remained the epicenter of the pandemic. It was so difficult hearing from friends and family members about people back home being infected with the virus left and right and many succumbing to the ugly virus as well.

I read many articles during this time about the virus affecting mainly older people, or mainly people with significant comorbidities or lung disease, etc. The unfortunate truth was that the largest disparity was the disproportionate amount of Black people that were hospitalized with the disease. It was not until maybe one to two months deep in the pandemic that the media began sharing this reality.

Health disparities are not to be blamed on the victims, but the blame is on the system. A system that is broken and has allowed systemic racism and bias affect how people of color are treated in the medical field. With the coronavirus pandemic, testing centers weren't as widely available, people of color were repeatedly turned away from being tested or hospitalized despite there being an inherent need, and resources were not evenly and widely distributed among the communities in which the majority of people of color live. Don't for one second believe the myths that health disparities occur for any other reason. This is the root of the bigger issue.

The Hippocratic oath states a lot of things and describes the duties of an ethically sound physician. There are many interpretations and revisions that have occurred over the past few centuries, so depending who you ask, you may get a different point of view. As a physician, you do vow to help people in the time of need. You do vow to use your knowledge and abilities to help and not harm patients. But nowhere in the oath does it say we are to sacrifice our lives and our families' lives by facing a highly infectious, deadly disease with inadequate protection. As I previously stated, we must be well to be able to care for other patients. If we do not take care of ourselves and our own health, we are of no good use to our patients.

The COVID-19 pandemic taught us many things about the world, healthcare, and ourselves. It taught us to band together during desperate times of need and to get creative to achieve daily tasks while practicing social distancing. Many of us healthcare workers: physicians, nurses, housekeeping, medical assistants, pharmacists, nursing assistants, technologists, etc., continued to work during these times. Many of us succumbed to the deadly virus. Many of us quit our jobs due to the unwillingness to sacrifice the health of our families. I respect each and every one of the decisions made by healthcare workers; as we all have different battles we face at home and no one should be made to feel guilty for their decision.

A career in medicine is going to take some sacrifice. The amount of sacrifice is up to you and the route you choose to go. Certain professions are more relaxed than others, or work less hours, or take less training and student loans, or make more money, etc. I urge you, dear reader, to truly pick the profession that is best for you including the lifestyle you plan to have. Just know that all professions will require sacrifice, but with hard work, determination, and genuine passion, it is all worth the journey when you have arrived at the dream.

Affirmation to recite*:* *My dreams are worth my sacrifices.*

Question: *When was a time that you took on a job that you later found out included more collateral duties than initially anticipated? How did you handle that situation? Did you continue working there or did you resign and change careers? If you stayed, what was it that urged you to stay?*

Afterword

Freshman year, I lived in a triple occupancy dorm room with two friends from high school, Brittany and Nita. We were all excited to be attending Michigan together and decided that rooming together would help us transition to a new unfamiliar environment. We all had different majors and rarely had classes together or even a similar schedule. Dinner was easier for us to link up at the end of the day since classes were all done.

"Are y'all ready to head to the cafeteria?" Nita asked Brittany and I as she entered our dorm room. It was just after 7 PM, but we typically ate late. We were nearing the end of our freshman year and had a routine, which usually involved later dinners. None of us were enthusiastic about the dorm food, but it kept us from gaining the freshman 15 we had feared.

"Sure!" I responded.

"I ate earlier today," Brittany stated. "I volunteered for an event back at our high school working with students who may want to go into kinesiology or sports medicine."

"Oh wow! That's cool! How was it?" I responded.

In high school, we had all taken many classes together as we were in all the honors or AP courses. Brittany had left before our junior year when her family moved to Texas. She didn't know some of our teachers from junior and senior year for that reason.

"It was great! It has been awhile since I walked the hallways. Everything looked pretty much the same though. Tamika, do you remember Dr. K?" She continued.

"Of course! He was one of my favorite teachers. He used to teach anatomy and physiology. I took his class as part of the medical academy. Does he remember me?" I questioned.

"Does he? He couldn't stop talking about you. He said you were always extremely talkative in class, so I knew he wasn't lying!" We laughed.

"Yea I got in trouble for socializing a time or two in his class, but it was hands down my favorite class. We did some cool dissections. It was the only class that felt like real medicine in high school. I couldn't wait to be a doctor after his class!" I reminisced.

"Yea he told me you were one of his favorite students beside being a chatty Kathy. He said you seemed genuinely interested in medicine and not just taking it to fulfill a prerequisite. I told him you decided not to go to medical school and were applying for the business school now." Brittany shared.

"What did he say to that?" I was perplexed.

"To be honest, he was upset. He kept talking about how great of a doctor and surgeon you would be. So when

I shared with him that you changed your career path, he couldn't understand why. He told me to tell you to rethink your decision," she replied.

"Ha! Good ole, Dr. K still giving me a hard time. I'm going to have to reach back out to him soon. I'm sure I'm not the first student of his that changed his or her mind and career path!"

◇◇◇◇◇◇◇◇◇◇◇◇◇◇◇◇◇◇◇◇◇◇◇◇◇◇◇◇◇◇◇◇◇◇◇

I remember this conversation like it was yesterday. When I was advised to change my major from medicine because it was an unlikely pathway for me, I didn't think much else about it. I continued down my path to take the prerequisites to apply for University of Michigan Ross School of Business. Although the classes were terribly boring and I wasn't doing exceptionally well, I had attributed it to be "part of the process". This was the first moment that I really stopped to think if I made the right decision.

Why did my 11th grade teacher care so much about me changing my major? Was he right? Was I making the right decision? Although I hadn't seen him in over a year and had not taken in class in two years, I felt guilty like I had let him down. It was an indescribable feeling. I later came to realize that the feeling was not because of how I made him feel, but rather my inner conscience telling me that I was making a huge mistake.

Once I snapped out of my daydreams after a couple days, I was back on track for applying to business school. It took a rejection letter for me to truly sit down and realize that this wasn't my calling. It made me think deeper as to why I had changed my major. Was it because I had lost interest in becoming a physician or was it because I was intimidated by the arduous journey I knew it would take to get there? As a generally stubborn person, it was unlike me to be so easily convinced, but in this situation my advisor telling me that medicine wasn't in my future hit differently.

After getting back on track for a pre-medicine curriculum and applying and successfully matriculating into medical school, Dr. K was one of the first people I reached out to. I couldn't wait to share the news that I was in fact going to be a doctor after all. He explained that he never once doubted me and my potential in getting to medical school and didn't understand why I had changed my mind. I had changed my mind due to my insecurities, self-doubt, and lack of appropriate mentorship. I was following the advice of someone who had known me for 20 minutes. All she saw was a 17-year-old Black girl with big dreams that to her small mind were unrealistic. She didn't know how ambitious, driven, and intelligent I was. She didn't know how hard of a worker I was. She didn't realize that I had dreamed of becoming a doctor since I could talk. Most importantly she didn't realize the deep impact of her negative energy and doubtful words.

I learned an important lesson pretty early on in my journey: not to expect someone else to see your vision. It was not like she had known me and mentored me for several years and watched my journey and truly felt it was not a good fit. She judged a book by its cover and to her I didn't look like a doctor. She also tried to apply the unfortunate statistics of how few minorities or "people like me" became physicians as reasoning as to why this goal was not going to be attainable. She was right that only few physicians were minorities, but she didn't dive into the reasoning behind it. My advisor didn't realize that one of the major reasons there are not enough of us is because we receive horrible discouraging advice from people like her that makes us rethink our goals and lifelong dreams. From that moment forward, I promised myself to keep pushing on the journey

Author Biography

Tamika knew at a young age that she wanted to pursue a career in medicine as a physician, but did not exactly know the steps it took to achieve her dream. Through unique opportunities, God-sent mentorship, hard work, and perseverance, Tamika was able to navigate the many obstacles necessary to achieve her childhood dream.

As a young doctor early in her career, Tamika found that the stereotypes and constant need to be validated did not disappear even after the 20 years of schooling she endured. One of many instances that highlighted this truth was when Tamika found herself on a plane, 30,000 feet in the air attempting to offer medical assistance to an unresponsive passenger, only to be denied access by crew members who did not believe Tamika was a doctor.

After sharing her story publicly, and gaining international media attention, Tamika was able to start a viral movement of hundreds of thousands of medical professionals all over the world who joined in solidarity by posting pictures of themselves with the hashtag #whatadoctorlookslike. By exemplifying the diversity amongst doctors, this movement was able to negate the myth that there is one prototype for what a doctor looks like. Beside starting an international conversation of bias in the workplace, Tamika's story became an integral part of diversity and inclusion training of schools and companies coast to coast. With her movement and executive meetings, she was able to implement policy change for a Fortune 100 company. Hundreds of published articles and news stories followed this viral movement for years to come. Dr. Cross' story was shared widely in the media, to include features in Forbes, CNN, *Essence Magazine*, BET, The Today Show, *The Washington Post*, and *The New York Times*.

Dr. Cross is a CEO of Serenity Women's Health and Medspa where she and her partner are both board-certified practicing Obstetrician and Gynecologists in the greater Houston area. Dr. Cross is a renowned speaker who has traveled across the country to speak on bias in the medical field, women's health topics, and the Black maternal mortality pandemic. She has garnered academic experience as an Assistant Professor as well as working in multiple healthcare systems, including one of the largest non-profit hospital systems in the state of Texas.

She has worked on quality improvement projects and committees to aid in securing a safe environment and experience for all patients. Dr. Cross has received numerous awards for her hard work and dedication to improving her communities. She was listed in the 2016 Becker Hospital Review Top 60 Most Powerful People in Healthcare alongside many healthcare moguls, including former President Barack Obama. Dr. Cross received United States Congressional Recognition for her community outreach. Her ability to identify obstacles and implement change for discrimination faced by minorities in medicine afforded her a University of Texas McGovern Medical School Faculty Senate Resolution as well.

While some may dismiss the experience of Dr. Cross on first glance, as a young Black female physician, she has numerable experiences throughout her journey, starting as a young girl, that have helped shape her into the young, Black, female professional, entrepreneur and physician she is today. She strives to be able to continue to use her experiences to empower our youth, aspiring physicians, or other minority professionals.

Appendix

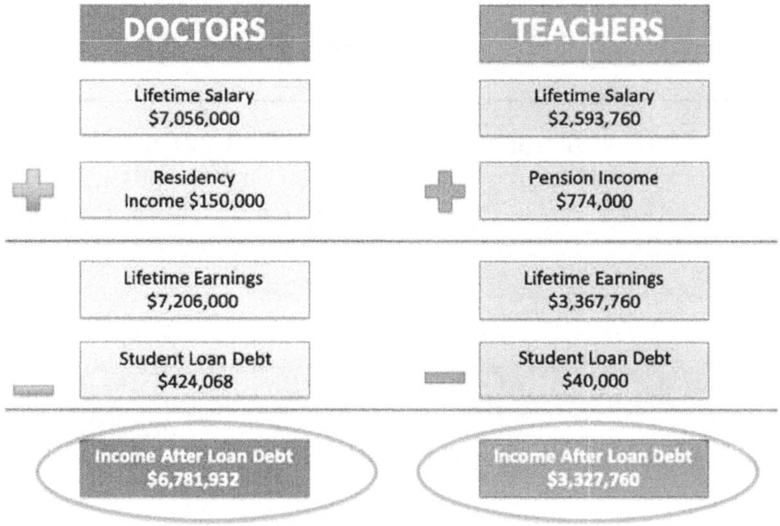

Figure 1

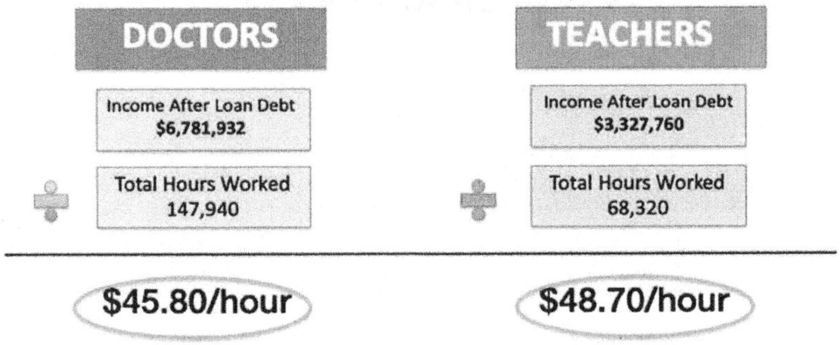

Figure 1.1

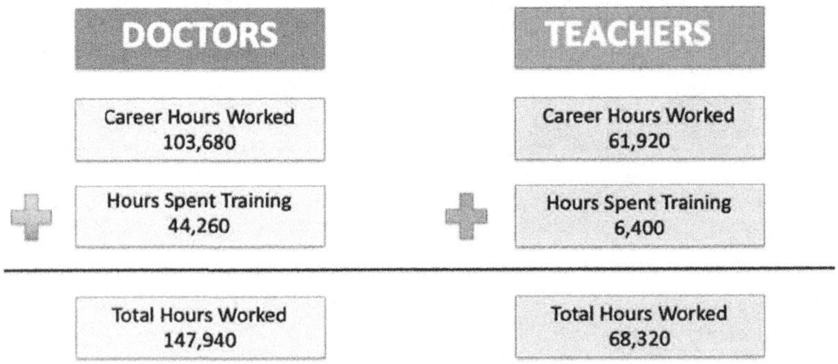

Figure 1.2

Made in the USA
Monee, IL
04 November 2026

67385383R00177